MANUAL OF
ULTRASONOGRAPHY

MANUAL OF ULTRASONOGRAPHY

KENNETH J. W. TAYLOR, M.D., Ph.D., F.A.C.P.
Professor of Radiology, Department of Diagnostic Radiology,
Yale University School of Medicine, New Haven, Connecticut

PAULA JACOBSON, R.T., R.D.M.S.
Diagnostic Sonographer, Department of Diagnostic Radiology,
Yale-New Haven Hospital, New Haven, Connecticut

CAROL A. TALMONT, R.T., R.D.M.S.
Diagnostic Sonographer, Department of Diagnostic Radiology,
Yale-New Haven Hospital, New Haven, Connecticut

RALPH WINTERS, R.T., R.D.M.S.
Diagnostic Sonographer, Department of Diagnostic Radiology,
Yale-New Haven Hospital, New Haven, Connecticut

DRAWINGS BY: CAROLINE R. TAYLOR, M.D.

CHURCHILL LIVINGSTONE
NEW YORK, EDINBURGH AND LONDON   1980

© Churchill Livingstone Inc. 1980

Distributed in the United Kingdom by Churchill Livingstone, Robert Stevenson House, 1-3 Baxter's Place, Leith Walk, Edinburgh EH1 3AF and by associated companies, branches and representatives throughout the world.

First published 1980

Printed in USA

ISBN 0 443 08053 4

7   6   5   4   3   2   1

Library of Congress Cataloging in Publication Data
Main entry under title:

Manual of ultrasonography.

    Bibliography: p.
    Includes index.
    1. Diagnosis, Ultrasonic.   I. Taylor,
Kenneth J. W., 1939-   II. Jacobson, Paula.
III. Talmont, Carol A.   IV. Winters, Ralph.
[DNLM: 1. Ultrasonics – Diagnostic use.
WB289 M294]
RC78.7.U4M35   616.07'54   79-23301
ISBN 0-443-08053-4

Preface

This book is intended as a companion volume to the *Atlas of Gray Scale Ultrasonography*. Whereas the *Atlas* shows a diversity of pathologic conditions, this manual concentrates on the scanning techniques employed at this institution to demonstrate normal anatomy as well as pathology.

Manual of Ultrasonography is primarily for the users of ultrasound equipment, including sonographers, residents and budding ultrasonologists. Under each organ system the relevant anatomy, physiology and clinical material are presented. This is mainly provided for the sonographer, and some sections will be too elementary for the physician. However, the remainder of the chapter should be valuable for physicians as well.

Ultrasound instrumentation is changing so rapidly that any text more than two years old becomes dated. I have therefore used the publication of this manual to update the physics and instrumentation chapters written for the *Atlas*. In addition, I have added a chapter on the applied physics involved in the production of artifacts which may produce pitfalls for the neophyte.

During the coming years, there is little doubt that most manual scanning will be replaced by various automated, real-time instruments. However, the scanning techniques described in this book will still be relevant, because the same scanning planes and approach angles must be used in manipulating the automated scanning heads.

We have considered aspiration and biopsy procedures in some detail, and this reflects the growing tendency at this institution to perform more and more invasive procedures under ultrasound guidance, in preference to fluoroscopy or computerized tomography. All too frequently we have seen patients with advanced pancreatic cancer and liver metastases subjected to laparotomy in the last few weeks of their lives, merely to confirm the diagnosis. Positive aspirations or biopsies can be obtained percutaneously in the vast majority of these patients, thereby avoiding unnecessary discomfort to the patient and the cost of futile surgery.

It is hoped that this book will provide the training sonographer with adequate material to pass the OB/GYN, abdominal and physics Registry examinations. I believe that it will also suffice for the Boards in Radiology. But more than this, we hope that it will provide a practical guide for those starting in the field of ultrasound.

KENNETH J. W. TAYLOR, M.D., Ph.D., F.A.C.P.
New Haven, 1979

Acknowledgments

We would like to thank our other sonographers and students, including Linda Alcebo, Eileen Barbieri, Lynne Gillooly, Linda Kostribiak, Karen Smith, Cheryl Smith and Andrea Testa, for their help in collecting the scans and for their comments on the manuscript. We would also like to thank Robin Charney and Cheryl Wilcox for their help in the preparation of the manuscript, and Robert Charney for Figure 15-1 A+B. Finally, we would like to thank the staff of Churchill Livingstone, especially Donna Balopole, Carole Baker and William Schmitt, for their patience and industry in the production of this book.

Contents

MANUAL OF ULTRASONOGRAPHY

1

Introduction to Basic Principles

KENNETH J. W. TAYLOR

DEFINITION OF BASIC TERMS

Frequency. Sound waves are mechanical oscillations which are transmitted by particles in
a gas, liquid or solid medium. Since a sound
wave is propagated by the movement of particles, a vacuum will not transmit sound. Infra-
sound is a term used for very low frequencies
below 16 cycles per second (cps), and such
frequencies are highly damaging. Audible
sound spans a frequency range from 16 to
about 16,000 cps, although children may hear
sounds up to 20,000 cps and the hearing
range of some animals extends even farther.
The term *ultrasound* refers to sound waves
beyond this audible range, and in medical applications a range of 1 to 10 million cps is employed.

Hertz indicates cycles per second, so
that the frequencies employed in medical applications are 1 to 10 Mega Hertz (MHz).

A Sound Wave is usually visualized as
a sinusoidal wave depicting the regular progress of a wave through the transmitting medium. Sound waves are variations in pressure,
and the sine wave represents these oscillations
which consist of a positive pressure wave followed by a negative pressure wave. The complete cycle of a positive and negative wave is a
wavelength, denoted as λ (Fig. 1-1).

Clearly, the product of the wavelength
and the number of waves per second
(frequency) is the distance traveled by the
wave in 1 second and this is the velocity (c).
Thus, we can write

$$F \times \lambda = c$$

The velocity of sound in any medium is constant at any given temperature. Thus, the frequency and the wavelength are reciprocally
related, that is, the higher the frequency, the
shorter the wavelength. Since resolution of

1

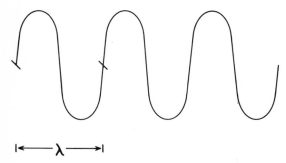

FIG. 1-1. The sound beam is characterized by a sine wave representing alternating compressions and rarefactions in the transmitting medium. The complete positive and negative phase constitutes one wavelength.

TABLE 1-1. POWER RATIOS AT SEVERAL DECIBEL LEVELS

dB	Power Ratio	Amplitude Ratio
6	3.98	2.0
20	100	31.6
30	1000	100.0
40	10,000 (10^4)	316.0
50	10^5	10^3
60	10^6	3.162
70	10^7	10^4
80 and so on	10^8 and so on	

any system is dependent on the wavelength, higher frequencies with shorter wavelengths allow better resolution.

Sound Intensity Notation. The term *sound intensity* refers to the power of the ultrasound wave. The units of absolute intensity are Watts/cm². Watts/cm² can be determined by measuring the pressure exerted by a sound wave. Thus, a sound intensity of 1 W/cm² exerts a pressure of 67 mg. Biological tissues, however, produce a very large range of acoustic echoes, and therefore it is more convenient to refer to a ratio of power levels. This is a logarithmic notation and is referred to as a *decibel* (dB). A decibel equals the ratio of the logarithm of one sound intensity to another. Thus, it may be mathmatically stated that 1 dB $= 10 \log_{10} \frac{p^1}{p^2}$, where p^1 and p^2 are the intensities of two ultrasound beams. Since this is a logarithmic power ratio, 20 dB refers to a power ratio of 10^2 or 100. Table 1-1 shows the power ratios corresponding to various decibel levels. From this table, it can be seen that the power ratios of 90 dB, which emanate from biological tissues, refer to a power ratio of 1 billion. To compare the size of an echo to the incident beam, it is often more convenient to measure amplitude rather than intensity. Intensity is proportional to the square of the amplitude, therefore the ratio in dB becomes

$$dB = 10 \log_{10} \left[\frac{A_1^2}{A_2^1} \right] = 20 \log_{10} \left[\frac{A_1}{A_2} \right]$$

where A_1 is the amplitude of the echo and A_2, that of the incident beam. The corresponding amplitude ratios are given in Table 1-1.

Huygen's Principle refers to the behavior of an ultrasound beam leaving a transducer. A transducer face is composed of a large number of small emitting elements from which sound waves spread out concentrically (Fig. 1-2A). Thus, if the transducer is very small compared to the wavelength, the beam will be widely divergent. When the transducer is larger, then the resultant beam is much less divergent and can be considered the sum of all the small sound sources (Fig. 1-2B).

PRODUCTION OF ULTRASOUND

We are familiar with the production of sound waves from vibrating vocal cords or stringed instruments. However, the frequencies used in medical diagnostic ultrasound are produced from a transducer, by the piezo-electric effect. A transducer is a means for converting one form of energy into another, in this instance electrical energy into mechanical sound waves. The piezo-electric effect was first described by Pierre and Jacques Curie in 1880. They observed that when certain naturally occurring crystals such as quartz underwent mechanical deformation, a potential difference developed across the two surfaces of the crystals. For reasons which will be considered later, quartz is not suitable for the diagnostic applications of ultrasound, but synthetic ceramics have been developed which are more efficient. A ceramic consists of charged particles which are linearly oriented by exposing them to a strong magnetic field during manufacture. The resulting ceramic can be cut into any shape depending upon the type of transducer to be manufactured. The ceramic most frequently used in diagnostic applications of ultrasound is composed of lead-zirconate and barium titanate, although there is continual work to develop different materials which are more efficient in converting electrical energy into sound energy. In the hand held transducer used in manual scanning techniques, the ceramic is in the form of a disc with its emitting surface curved to produce a focused beam. Any given ceramic has a resonant frequency at which it will produce ultrasound most efficiently, and this frequency depends on the thickness of the ceramic.

Ultrasound at the frequencies used in medical diagnosis is therefore produced by the piezo-electric effect from a ceramic. When a rapidly alternating electric current is applied across a ceramic at its resonant frequency, an ultrasound beam is produced with maximum efficiency for the conversion of electric energy to acoustic energy. As the driving frequency varies from the resonant frequency of the transducer, the efficiency of this energy conversion decreases markedly. However, the transducer will resonate not only at its fundamental frequency but also at its 3rd, 5th, 7th harmonics etc. with decreasing efficiency. In practice the variation in transducer efficiency with driving frequency is only relevant when continuous (CW) wave ultrasound is used. In the imaging systems currently under consideration, a very short pulse of ultrasound is used, (for reasons which will be discussed later) and in these applications wide frequency ranges are used, rather than a single pure frequency. This range is called the *bandwidth.*

Bandwidth of an Ultrasound Signal refers to the frequency spectrum. When a continuous wave of ultrasound is produced, a single pure frequency can be emitted. However, when a ceramic is hit with a single very short electrical impulse, a wide variety of different frequencies are emitted, so that there is a wide frequency spectrum or bandwidth (Fig. 1-3).

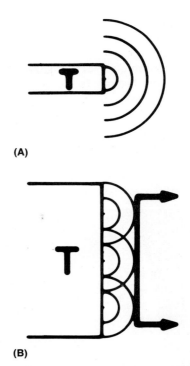

(A)

(B)

FIG. 1-2. The shape of an ultrasound beam emitted from any given transducer is dictated by Hugyen's principle. **(A)** When the transducer (T) is small compared with the wavelength, sound waves spread out concentrically and produce a wide beam. **(B)** When the transducer (T) face is large relative to the wavelength, the behavior of the ultrasound beam can be considered as the sum of small sound sources which are linearly arranged. As the beam spreads out concentrically from each of them, the overall beam profile is a parallel wave front the width of the transducer face.

Although in pulse echo techniques we conventionally do talk about a nominal 3MHz frequency, since the attenuation of ultrasound increases almost linearly with frequency (see below), the ultrasound bandwidth actually changes as it passes through tissues because the higher frequencies are attenuated. Because of the attenuation of high frequencies, claims of imaging the entire liver using a 7 MHz transducer are fallacious. Such a transducer may have a frequency spectrum from 4–10 MHz, and the higher frequencies are rapidly attenuated by passage through tissues. Thus the deeper tissues are being imaged only by the lower frequencies remaining after absorption of the higher ones.

Pulse Length

A brief consideration of the principles in short pulse-echo techniques demonstrates the importance of the brevity of the pulse for optimal resolution. We can consider imaging at a frequency of 3 MHz when the wavelength is 0.5 mm: if ten cycles of ultrasound were emitted, this train of pulses would extend for a distance of 5.0 mm (Fig. 1-4). If this pulse of ultrasound hits a thin interface, part of this

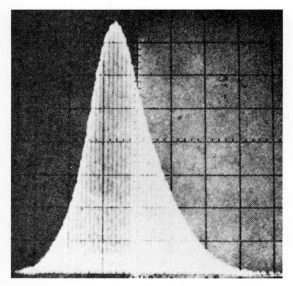

FIG. 1-3. Frequency spectrum of wide bandwidth transducer. The nominal frequency refers to the peak, but considerable frequency ranges are present, both below and above that peak.

energy is reflected along the same path as the original beam. This returning echo is a sound pressure wave which causes slight mechanical deformation of the ceramic as it impinges on the transducer face. This results in an electrical pulse as a result of the piezo-electric properties of the ceramic. If the original pulse were 10 cycles (5 mm) in length, the shortest echo would be 5.0 mm, and a thin interface could only be represented by a minimum distance of 5 mm. This would lead to a severe degradation in the resolution of the ultrasound imaging system in the plane of the transducer beam, which is called the axial plane. The lateral res-

olution is the plane parallel to the transducer face and is considered later (pp. 12-14).

From these considerations it should be apparent that the ultrasound pulse should be as short as possible to optimize the axial resolution. The shortest ultrasound pulse possible is a single sound wave cycle (0.5 mm at a frequency of 3 MHz). In practice it is difficult to achieve this extreme brevity since transducers are similar to bells when they are struck, and tend to produce a prolonged peal of sound. However, an ultrasound transducer can be damped similar to the way in which a peal of bells can be silenced by holding the bell. In the manufacture of ultrasound transducers, damping to produce a very short pulse, is achieved by "backing" the transducer with an absorbant substance such as Araldite. Thus, the after ringing of the transducer can be minimized following excitation by an electric pulse. (Fig. 1-5)

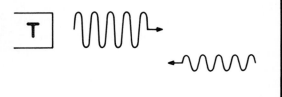

FIG. 1-4. Effect of pulse length on axial resolution. If a train of 10 sound wave cycles is emitted, the length of the pulse is 5 mm, the length of the echo is 5 mm and the axial resolution is 5 mm. To achieve good axial resolution, the length of the pulse must be as short as possible, which in practice proves to be 2 or 3 cycles, lasting approximately one microsecond.

Achieving a very short ultrasonic pulse also depends on the choice of the material for the transducer. As mentioned above, quartz is not used for medical diagnostic devices because it tends to ring for many cycles after excitation. Any material which produces a long train of sound waves in response to a single energizing electrical pulse is said to have a high Q. In fact quartz has a Q of approximately 1500, indicating that it produces some 1500 cycles in response to a single energizing electrical pulse. In comparison, the ceramics used in medical diagnostic devices have a mechanical Q around 50, that is, only 50 cycles of sound are produced in response to a single energizing pulse of electrical power. This Q is substantially reduced by heavy damping from the Araldite on the back surface of the transducer. In fact, the damping results in an ultrasound pulse lasting approximately 1 microsecond (μs) (one millionth of a second), and comprises 2 to 3 sound wave cycles of rapidly diminishing amplitude (Fig. 1-5). Effectively, therefore, the pulse emitted from these instruments is less than a microsecond in length and produces resolution around 1 mm in the axial plane of the transducer.

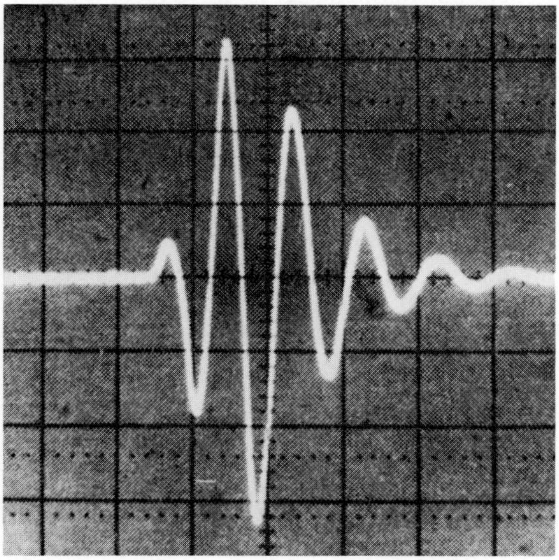

FIG. 1-5. Oscilloscope tracing of short pulse consisting of two or three sound wave cycles of rapidly diminishing amplitude due to heavy damping of the transducer.

Behavior of the Ultrasound Beam at Interfaces

The behavior of an ultrasound beam is similar to that of a light beam in that it may be reflected, refracted or diffracted at interfaces between different media. At the junction of two media of different acoustic properties, referred to as acoustic impedance, an ultrasound beam

may be reflected depending on the difference in acoustic impedance between the two media and the angle of incidence (the angle at which the beam hits the interface). In biological tissues, with the exception of air/tissue and soft tissue/bone interfaces, the differences in acoustic impedance are rather slight so that only a small component of the ultrasound beam will be returned at each interface. Most of the energy passes into the deeper tissues and again, is reflected at other interfaces.

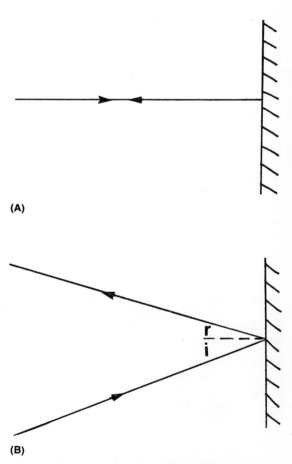

(A)

(B)

FIG. 1-6. Specular reflectors. **(A)** When the beam is at normal incidence to a mirror-like reflector, virtually all the energy is returned to the transducer. **(B)** When the sound beam is incident on a mirror-like surface, it is reflected such that the angle of incidence equals the angle of reflection and virtually none of the beam returns to the transducer.

Types of Reflectors in Biological Tissues

When considering the interaction of the ultrasound beam with biological tissues at least three different types of reflectors must be considered.

Specular Reflectors are analogous to a beam of light striking a mirror. At such an interface, the beam is reflected such that the angle of incidence equals the angle of reflection (Fig. 1-6B). This type of reflector is often the only one considered in the physics of ultrasound in books on diagnostic techniques, and yet it is probably the least important. Specular echoes are very large, that is, a substantial portion of the beam may be reflected, and the amplitude of the returned echo is highly dependent upon the orientation of the beam to the reflector. We can see from Figure 1-6 that the reflected beam will not return to the transducer unless the beam is perpendicular to the reflector. Specular reflectors are therefore characterized by high amplitude with extreme dependence on angle of orientation. In biological tissues, reflectors such as the diaphragm, fetal skull or vertebral column are all specular reflectors. The sonographer can investigate the nature of specular reflectors by directing an ultrasound beam onto one of these interfaces and inspecting the A-scan. If the beam is normal (perpendicular to the interface), a large echo will be seen on the A-scan (Fig. 1-7A),

and as the transducer is rocked so that the beam is at an acute angle to the interface, a much smaller echo will be seen from it on the A-scan (Fig. 1-7B).

Backscattered Echoes are probably of considerable importance in clinical imaging. However, a comprehensive theory has not yet been developed for the behavior of a sound beam at these reflectors. They are structures whose size is similar to that of the wavelength, so that their echogenicity may vary at different frequencies. An important facet of this type of reflector is that it results in echoes with little variation in angle of incidence. This has important implications for the display of soft tissue parenchyma. We have seen that the amplitude of specular echoes, for example, is highly dependent upon angle of incidence. In contrast, the amplitude of back-scattered, low level echoes arising from the parenchyma of soft tissues, is independent of angle of attack but is dependent on the type and amount of the reflector. Thus, if high level echoes are seen from within the soft tissues, it is not due to the random orientation of the beam but implies that there has been a change within the consistency of that tissue. As we shall describe later, deposition of fibrous tissue or fat particles is a common cause of increased echo amplitude from the soft tissue parenchyma.

Rayleigh Scattering, named after the

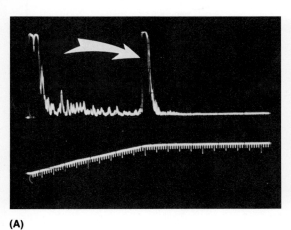 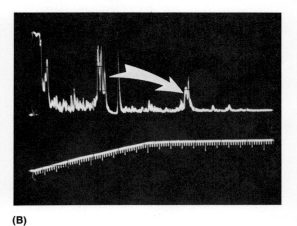

(A) **(B)**

FIG. 1-7. Variation of amplitude of specular reflector with angle of incidence. **(A)** A large specular echo (arrowed) from the diaphragm when the beam is at normal incidence. **(B)** When the beam is moved to an acute angle to the diaphragm, the amplitude of the returned echo is much smaller.

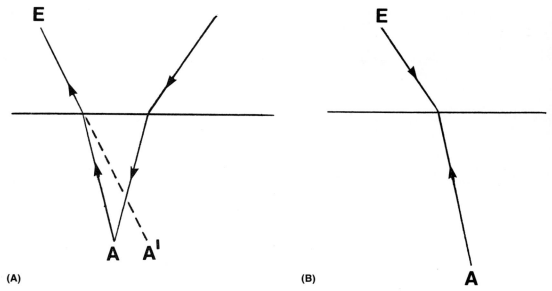

FIG. 1-8. Refraction. **(A)** When the reflector (A) is illuminated by a beam which is not coincident with that returning to the eye (E) or transducer, the beam is refracted but the eye assumes that the beam has travelled in a straight line, so that the reflector (A) is considered to be in the position of (A'). **(B)** When the illuminating beam is refracted to the same extent as the returned echo, there is no distortion in the position of A. This is the arrangement in diagnostic ultrasound scanning in the reflective mode.

British Physicist, Lord Rayleigh, has been well described. Rayleigh reflectors are very small compared with the wavelength of the ultrasound beam. In biological systems, red blood cells (7μ in diameter) give rise to Rayleigh scattering when ultrasound has a wavelength of 0.15 – 1.5 mm. (1 – 10 MHz). Such reflectors have a strong frequency dependence since the amplitude of returning echoes varies with the fourth power of the frequency. Thus, when the frequency is doubled from 1 to 2 MHz, the amplitude of the returning echo will be increased by a factor of 16 (2^4). In the use of sonar, no strong dependence on frequency change is observed, so it appears that this mechanism may be of little importance.

Diffraction and Refraction

Diffraction is a phenomenon which involves bending of an ultrasound beam around a small reflector. This has some importance in the diagnosis of gallstones as detailed later (p. 119). For diffraction to occur, the reflector must be smaller than the beam-width. The

reflector will be "seen" by the transducer since it produces an echo which will be received and amplified. However, the beam diffracts around the reflector and continues as a coherent beam.

Refraction refers to the bending of an ultrasound beam at the interface between media of different acoustic properties (Figs. 1-8A – B). It will be recalled that the phenomenon of refraction of light produces distortion of any object which is partially immersed in water (Fig. 1-8A). Refraction will not, however, produce distortion of an image in sonar imaging systems. This is because the same transducer is used as a source of the ultrasound beam and the receiver of the returned beam. Thus, if the beam is bent during its course to the reflector, the echo will be bent back in the opposite direction (Fig. 1-8B). Thus, there will be no distortion of the object. However, in experimental systems in which ultrasound transmission imaging is attempted, there will be distortion. This is one of the problems in trying to image an organ such as the breast by transmission imaging. The ultrasound beam is

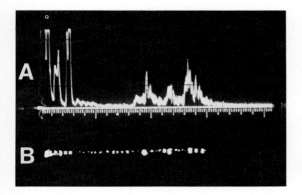

bent on entering the breast and on leaving it. Using this transmission ultrasonic imaging system, it cannot be assumed that the ultrasound beam has traveled in a straight line.

Generation of A, B and M-mode Scans

We have defined the way in which a very short pulse of ultrasound is emitted from an ultrasonic transducer and the necessity for extreme brevity of the pulse. We have also considered the mechanisms by which such an ultrasound

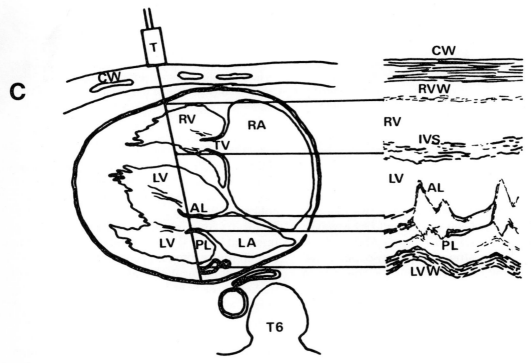

FIG. 1-9. **(A)** A-mode scan across the liver. The amplitude of the echoes as seen on the A-scan is proportional to the change of acoustic properties at each interface. **(B)** Brightness modulated line corresponding to the A-scan. **(C)** Schema to show the M-mode scan. An ultrasound beam is passed across the heart in the anatomical position shown in the schema. The beam transects the right ventricle (RV), left ventricle (LV) and is incident upon both anterior (AL) and posterior (PL) mitral valve leaflets. The interventricular septum (IVS) can be seen between the ventricular cavities, the right ventricular wall (RVW) is seen anteriorly, and the chest wall (CW) intervenes between the heart and the transducer (T). The posterior left ventricular wall (LVW) is seen, as are the atria (RA and LA). The tricuspid valve is designated TV. The line of ultrasonic data is brightness modulated, and then the tracing is moved in time either mechanically or electrically, which results in a recording of the position of various heart structures as they move in time. Thus, an M-mode tracing is a two-dimensional recording—one spatial and one temporal—and the gradient of any line on the M-mode recording will be the velocity with which the structure moves, since it is the rate at which the structures are moving in time.

beam can be reflected at different interfaces within the tissues. We now consider how these echoes are converted into images used in A, B and M-mode scanning.

A-Mode (Amplitude Modulation) As the short pulse of ultrasound traverses biological tissues, multiple small interfaces are encountered. At each of these interfaces, a small fraction of that energy is returned along the path of the incident ultrasound beam towards the transducer. Each of these fractions of the original energy sequentially hits the transducer face and produces an electrical potential by the reverse piezo-electric effect. Thus, in response to a single short pulse of ultrasound energy, a string of pulses is received back at the transducer. The first ones are from the superficial tissues, and the subsequent ones from deeper tissues. All these echoes can be shown on an oscilloscope as blips or deflections from the base line. The bigger the echo which is received, the larger the blip on the oscilloscope tube so that this display is amplitude modulated (A-mode). A-mode is a single line of information in space (Fig. 1-9A).

B-Mode (Brightness Modulation) B-mode is by far the most widely used presentation for ultrasound images and consists of two spatial dimensions. It is therefore a spatial tomogram. A B-mode scan is produced from a large series of A-scans by brightness modulation (Fig. 1-9A & B).

The A-scan is first converted into a series of dots in which the larger the echo, the brighter the dot. The transducer is now moved manually in a second plane, and the echoes of the original A-scan are held on the screen to build up a two dimensional image. Other means can be found for mechanically or electronically moving the ultrasound beam but all these systems, the so-called real-time systems, result in the formation of B-scan tomograms.

M-Mode (Time Position Mode) M-mode or time position mode is most widely used in imaging the heart to demonstrate movement. M-mode has been complemented by real-time imaging, which is essentially a three-dimen-

sional display, that is, two dimensions moving in time. In M-mode, the brightness scan shown in Figure 1-9C is written on paper which is moved, producing a two-dimensional scan. In this scan, one dimension is movement in space and the other is time. Thus, it records the movements of all structures in a single line along the ultrasound beam, and it records their movements with time. At an interface such as the pulsating heart walls, an undulating line is written on the moving paper.

ACOUSTIC PROPERTIES OF TISSUES

Biological tissues have a number of different properties which affect the interaction between them and an ultrasound beam. We now consider some of the important properties of biological tissues.

TABLE 1-2. VELOCITIES OF ULTRASOUND IN VARIOUS MEDIA AND SOFT TISSUES

Material	Velocity (m/sec)
Air	331
Water	1,430
Fat	1,450
Liver	1,550
Kidney	1,560
Blood	1,570
Skull Bone	4,080

Velocity of Sound Although there are wide differences in the velocity of sound in air, bone and soft tissue, there are very small differences between the velocity in various soft tissues (Table 1-2). For example, the velocity of sound in air is approximately 330 meters per second (m/s) and in bone approximately 4000 m/s. In soft tissue, the velocity is approximately 1500 m/s with only small differences between different components of soft tissue.

Density As with differences in velocity, there are rather large differences in the densities of soft tissue and bone and soft tissue and air.

Obviously, the density of air is very small compared to that of soft tissue, while the density of bone is high. However, the differences of density in soft tissues are relatively slight.

Acoustic Impedance Acoustic impedance is the product of the velocity of sound in a medium and the density of that medium. As has already been considered, the differences in velocity and density between soft tissues are small, and so differences in acoustic impedance are similarly small, generally amounting to less than 5 percent. However, while the the differences in acoustic impedance between soft tissues are relatively small, those between soft tissue and air, and between soft tissue and bone, are large.

The amount of ultrasound energy reflected at an interface between materials of different acoustic properties is dependent on the difference in acoustic impedance. The amplitude of the reflected component can be quantitated by the expression:

$$R = \frac{Z^1 - Z^2}{Z^1 + Z^2}$$

where Z^1 and Z^2 are the acoustic impedances of the materials forming the interface. Z equals the product of C (velocity of sound in that medium) and p (density of that medium). The low density of air and the high density of bone account for the large differences in their acoustic impedance (Table 1-3). This simple equation also accounts for the extremely destructive effect of air on ultrasound scans. Air has a low density and low velocity of sound,

so its acoustic impedance is low compared to that of soft tissues, in which the density approaches unity and the velocity is 1500 m/s. This implies that there would be a large reflection of sound at soft tissue/air interfaces, and the amplitude of this reflected component approaches 99.9 percent. Similarly, because of the high velocity and high density of bone, there will be substantial reflection at soft tissue/bone interfaces.

Bulk Modulus As we have considered, the differences in velocity and density in soft tissues appear to be rather small, and there is difficulty in accounting for the echogenicity of soft tissue. However, the differences in the acoustic properties of soft tissue become simpler to understand if these are considered in terms of their bulk modulus, rather than in terms of density or velocity differences. The important differences in bulk modulus were first pointed out by Fields and Dunn in 1975. The bulk modulus of the medium refers to its elasticity, or its rigidity (lack of elasticity). When a structure serves as a support for soft tissues, it must be more rigid than the surrounding soft tissues which are supported by it. The supporting tissues also include collagen, elastin and other supporting tissues of the fibrous skeleton. The expression relating acoustic impedance to the amplitude of the reflected component can be written:

$$R \simeq \frac{B_1^{1/2} - B_2^{1/2}}{B_1^{1/2} + B_2^{1/2}}$$

(Where B_1 and B_2 are the bulk moduli of the media forming the interface). Fields and Dunn (1975) pointed out that the bulk modulus of collagen and related fibrous proteins was approximately 10,000 times greater than that of surrounding tissues, so that differences in bulk modulus can form the basis for relatively large differences in acoustic impedance.

In practice it does appear that collagen and other similar interfaces are effective sites of echo formation. Probably the echogenicity of liver and kidney results from the collagen contained therein. However, collagen interfaces are not the only ones that are important

TABLE 1-3. CHARACTERISTIC ACOUSTIC IMPEDANCE OF VARIOUS MEDIA AND SOFT TISSUES

Material	Acoustic Impedance
Air	0.0001
Fat	1.38
Water	1.50
Blood	1.61
Kidney	1.62
Liver	1.65
Muscle	1.70
Skull Bone	7.80

in clinical imaging. As referred to previously, it appears that the deposition of fat, as for example in fatty infiltration, also increases the echogenicity of an organ. Thus, it appears that there are multiple mechanisms whereby echoes are produced from soft tissues, and important among these are collagen and fatty particles.

Attenuation Attenuation is the sum of acoustic energy losses resulting from absorption, scattering and reflection; in normal tissues approximately 80 percent of the loss of sound energy is by absorption with 20% being lost by scatter and reflection. However, when the number of scatterers is increased, as for example in a fatty infiltrated organ, the resulting loss of energy due to scattering becomes increased, and there will be abnormally high attenuation by such tissues. Acoustic energy is also heavily attenuated at soft tissue/air and soft tissue/bone interfaces because of the large differences in acoustic impedance at these interfaces. Gallstones are a further rigid interface, which like bone, will produce marked attenuation so that only a fraction of the incident energy is transmitted through the stone. This results in an acoustic shadow which is considered later (pp. 37–38).

As with all energy forms, attenuation is an exponential phenomenon, that is, it increases with the square of the distance traveled. Thus, when the distance is doubled the attenuation is increased by a factor of four. Attenuation of ultrasound increases linearly with the frequency of the ultrasound beam. Thus, at a frequency of 2 MHz, attenuation is approximately twice that of 1 MHz. The published values for attenuation vary widely, but reliable estimates indicate that this is approximately 1 dB/MHz/cm for a round trip. Thus at the frequency of 3 MHz, attenuation over a distance of 15 cm from the transducer amounts to approximately 45 dB.

Time Gain Control (TGC) Time gain control is the electronic compensation for tissue attenuation. Since attenuation is exponential, time gain control is also exponential. That is, an echo that comes from twice the distance is given four times the amplification so that a similar echo amplitude emanates from similar

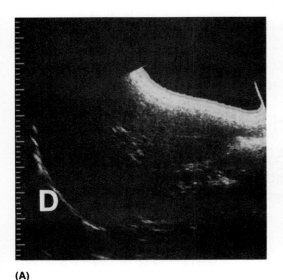
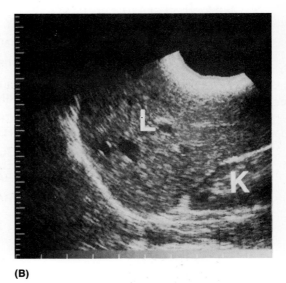

(A)   **(B)**

FIG. 1-10. Effect of addition of time-gain control. **(A)** B-scan through the liver and right kidney without addition of TGC. Notice that the liver substance is not written beyond the first few centimeters, while the diaphragm (D) being a large specular reflector, is still apparent. **(B)** B-scan of liver and right kidney after addition of TGC. Notice there is a homogeneous texture throughout the whole of the liver (L), and the right kidney (K) is also clearly visible. This indicates that there is correct compensation for tissue attenuation.

reflectors independent of the distance from the transducer and the effects of attenuation. At the present, the TGC must be set by an experienced ultrasonologist and improper TGC setting can produce an abnormal parenchymal pattern or even simulate a tumor or abscess cavity.

The importance of correct TGC is demonstrated in the following figures: Figure 1-10A shows an A-scan through the liver without the addition of TGC. Note that there is rapid attenuation of the ultrasound beam and that the deep parts of the organ are not displayed. The addition of proper TGC (Fig. 1-10B) elevates the amplitude of distal echoes to a similar height as those from the superficial parts of the liver; that is, the effects of attenuation have been overcome by selective amplification of the far echoes. Since tissue attenuation increases almost linearly with frequency, any change of frequency during scanning implies that the TGC must be readjusted.

RESOLUTION OF AN ULTRASOUND IMAGING SYSTEM

The resolution of an ultrasound imaging system in the two planes of the tomogram must be considered separately. The axial plane is the plane of the ultrasound beam, and the resolution is dependent upon the brevity of the ultrasound pulse. Transient excitation of the ceramic combined with heavy damping produces a pulse of about 1 microsecond in duration and an axial resolution of around 1 mm.

The lateral resolution is largely dependent on beam width, and therefore varies at different distances from the transducer and with the frequency. In the transducers commonly used in clinical practice, a realistic lateral resolution is around 3 mm in the narrowest part of the focal zone and perhaps 10 mm in the far zone. Examination of any ultrasound tomogram through a fairly homogeneous organ such as the liver gives some idea of the

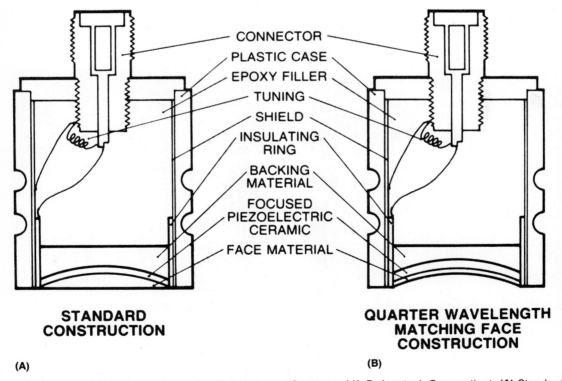

STANDARD
CONSTRUCTION

QUARTER WAVELENGTH
MATCHING FACE
CONSTRUCTION

CONNECTOR
PLASTIC CASE
EPOXY FILLER
TUNING
SHIELD
INSULATING RING
BACKING MATERIAL
FOCUSED PIEZOELECTRIC CERAMIC
FACE MATERIAL

(A)

(B)

FIG. 1-11. Construction of transducers in clinical usage. (Courtesy of K. B. Aerotech Corporation). **(A)** Standard construction. **(B)** Quarter wave matching layer.

resolution if we assume that the reflectors within such an organ are similar throughout.

FOCUSING THE ULTRASOUND BEAM

Since the lateral resolution of an ultrasound imaging system depends upon the beam width, the ability to focus the beam and thereby reduce its lateral dimensions is important. Ideally, a pencil-thin beam of ultrasound is required so that there is good resolution throughout the field. Unfortunately there is no means by which this ideal can be approached, and all attempts to do so represent a compromise. An ultrasound beam can be highly focused to produce a fairly narrow focal region, but this results in a very limited focal zone with wide dispersion of the beam, both before and after the focal region. A compromise, therefore, consists of a relatively narrow beam for the longest focal depth possible. In the manual transducers currently employed, this relatively weak focusing of the ultrasound beam is produced by using a curved ceramic (Fig. 1-11A). The distance of the focal zone can be selected according to the engineering of the ceramic face and the frequency involved. However, the configuration of the focal zone is fixed for any one transducer, so that a number of different transducers are required for the satisfactory examination of any particular patient when organs at different depths from the transducer are of particular interest. Beam profiles of transducers in common clinical practice are seen in Figures 1-12 A & B. It should be noted that when a 19 mm transducer face is used, the beam emerging from the transducer face is wide. The beam width does not approach less than 5 mm until approximately 5 cm away from the transducer face. Thus, the lateral resolution of a commonly used transducer does not start to reach an acceptable width for some distance from the transducer face, and the effect of the distant focal zone has important implications for optimal imaging (pp. 40–41). The focal zone of the transducer has important implications for the echo amplitude from similar reflectors. Figure 1-12B shows the echo amplitude from a standard reflector at various distances from the transducer face. In the focal zone, the echo amplitude is high within the narrow confines of the focus. This variation in echo amplitude is apparent on clinical scans. These considerations demonstrate the problems of attempting to quantitate echo amplitude from organs (now available on commercial equipment on A-scan analysis) unless these beam width effects are taken into account. In the highly sophisticated phased array systems which are becoming commercially available, the focal zone of the transducer can be varied, and this is known as dynamic focusing. These systems are considered later (pp. 27–29).

QUARTER WAVE MATCHING LAYERS

Quarter wave matching layers represent a new improvement in ultrasound technology, which has led to some prolongation of the focal zone but predominantly in increased sensitivity of a transducer. There is increased efficiency with which ultrasound energy is coupled into the patient and out again to the transducer. This is achieved by the addition of a plastic material to the front of the ceramic (Fig. 1-11B). The acoustic impedance of this material is halfway between the acoustic impedance of the ceramic and that of the patient's body, and it can be shown that this substantially increases the amount of energy coupled into and out of the patient. The thickness of this plastic material is equal to one-quarter the wavelength for the reason shown schematically in Figure 1-13A–C.

One-quater wavelength traverses the matching layer simultaneously with a returning echo which is in phase with the emitted beam. Because these are in phase, the amplitude of the two will be increased due to constructive interference. Thus, the quarter wave matching layer increases the energy transferred to and from the patient.

SIGNAL PROCESSING

The signal processing involved in commercially produced ultrasound imaging systems underwent a revolution in 1974 with the advent of gray-scale systems. This system differs from the bistable systems previously employed, in which either an echo had sufficiently large amplitude to be recorded or it was below the given threshold and was not recorded on the cathode-ray tube (CRT) at all. A bistable scan is shown in Figure 1-14A and compared with a gray-scale scan in Figure 1-14B. It is obvious that the bistable scan discards an enormous amount of quantitative information on echo amplitude and that echoes of many different sizes above the critical threshold are displayed at uniform intensity.

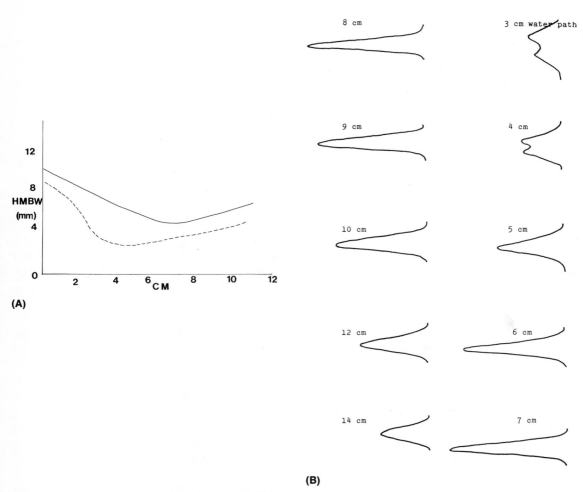

FIG. 1-12. **(A)** Beam profile of two transducers in common clinical usage. The X axis is the distance from the transducer face. The beam width (Y axis) characterized here is half the maximum intensity and above (HMBW). The continuous upper line is a 2.25 MHz, 13 mm face unfocused transducer, and the lower dotted line, a 2.25 MHz, 13 mm face medium internal focus transducer. Note the very wide beam width close to the transducer face and the divergence of the beam beyond the focal zone. These three regions, before, at the focal zone and beyond it can be referred to as the near zone, focal zone and far zone respectively. **(B)** Beam intensity profiles at various distances from the transducer face (2.25 MHz, 13 mm face, medium internal focus). At 3 cm from the face in the near zone, the intensity profile is peaked and this results in multiple echoes from a single reflector. All profiles were obtained from a standard reflector, and yet the largest echo is obtained at 7 and 8 cm because this coincides with the focal zone of the transducer. Echo amplitude is extremely dependent upon the focusing characteristics of the transducer, and the extent of the focal zone is limited (Courtesy of K.B. Aerotech Corp).

Equally unsatisfactory is the failure to register the many small echoes coming from within soft tissue parenchyma. Thus, essentially only large specular echoes were displayed, while the clinically important backscattered soft tissue echoes were lost; cystic lesions could be diagnosed by scanning the patient at increasing gain, but subtle soft tissue textural differences were entirely lost.

GRAY-SCALE SYSTEMS

The major problem to be solved in signal processing and display of gray-scale systems originated in the enormous dynamic range which emanates from biological tissues. In the typical clinical scan, a range of approximately 90 dB exists between the size of the smallest and largest echoes from tissues. It should be recalled that this represents a power ratio of one billion to one. This vast dynamic range is somewhat reduced by the addition of time gain control, since many of these echoes are very small because of tissue attenuation. The addition of approximately 45 dB of TGC reduces the dynamic range of the signal to be displayed to 45 dB. This contrasts markedly with a dynamic range of most display systems, including cathode ray tubes and scan converters, which is between 15–20 dB. It is because of the limited range of these systems that only a

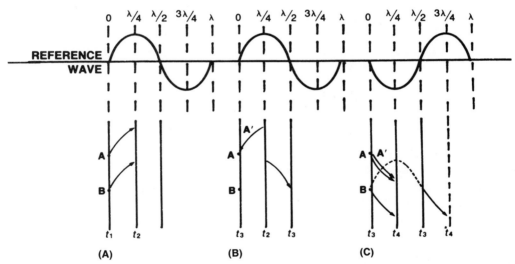

FIG. 1-13. A representation of what occurs within the facing material when ultrasonic waves are propagated through it. Points A and B are two out of an infinite number of point sources of ultrasonic waves on the piezoelectric ceramic. In **(A)** ultrasonic waves are initiated by point sources A and B at time t_1. At time t_2, the waves have reached the interface between the facing material and the body. The reflection/transmission phenomena occurs at time t_2. In **(B)** wave A is reflected (A′) and wave B is transmitted at the interface. At time t_3, both of the waves have travelled one-half of a wave-length if the face material is one-quarter wavelength thick. That is, wave A′ has travelled one-quarter wavelength to the face and one-quarter wavelength back to the ceramic. Wave B has travelled one-quarter wavelength to the face and one-quarter wavelength beyond. In **(C)** at time t_3, point source A and B are at the position corresponding to one-half wavelength on the reference ultrasonic wave. (It is important to note that for the very short time intervals involved from t_1 to t_4, the ceramic may be considered to be generating ultrasonic waves continuously.) At time t_4 the reflected wave A′, the new wave front generated by point A, and the new wave front generated by point B arrive at the transducer face/body interface in phase producing signal reinforcement. This is a continuous process, as some ultrasonic energy is always reflected each time the wave front encounters an interface. It is also important to note that the same effect also occurs when the echoes from body structures impinge upon the transducer. The waves reflected within the face undergo the same phase reversals and signal reinforcement into the ceramic (Courtesy of K.B. Aerotech Corporation).

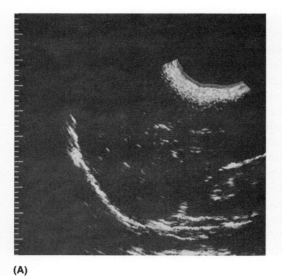

(A)

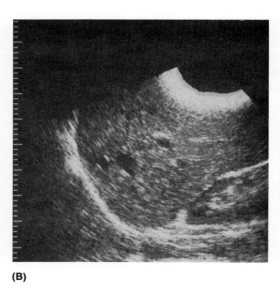

(B)

FIG. 1-14. **(A)** Bistable scan of the liver and right kidney (Fig. 1-14A) compared with **(B)** a gray-scale scan. Notice that the gray-scale technology allows the parenchyma of soft tissues to be imaged, so that small defects within it, due to small liver vessels, are clearly seen. Other details include the intrahepatic bile vessels, perirenal fat and the renal medulla. Thus, gray-scale display results in greatly improved visualization of important anatomic detail.

small segment of these signals can be displayed.

The term *gray-scale* refers to the selective amplification of low level echoes which originate from within soft tissues and display these echoes at the expense of larger echoes. A schema of this type of signal processing is shown in Figure 1-15. This is known as the compression amplification characteristic of gray-scale imaging systems. A limited dynamic range of the display system is shown on the Y-axis, while the large dynamic range put into the system is shown on the X-axis. This schema shows that most of the display is devoted to lower level echoes, which are therefore preferentially displayed. The larger echoes, which are specular in origin are increasingly compressed. The importance of this type of signal processing is the retention and display of the low level echoes which are backscattered from within soft tissue parenchyma. We have already considered that the amplitude of specular echoes is largely dependent upon the orientation of the beam to any particular reflector, and therefore the absolute amplitude of the reflectors is random. It is because of the

nature of these reflectors that the compression of this type of data leads to little loss of clinically important information.

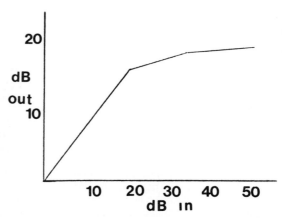

FIG. 1-15. Type of compression amplification schema employed in gray-scale imaging. The large dynamic range (dB in) of echoes returned from biological tissues must be compressed into the limited dynamic range of the display system (dB out). Most of the display is devoted to the lower level echoes from the parenchyma, while the larger, predominantly specular echoes, are increasingly compressed.

PRE-SIGNAL PROCESSING

Pre-signal processing refers to the use of a compression amplication curve which is different from that shown schematically in Figure 1-15. Such a curve may be linear, sigmoid or other shape; examples are shown in Figure 1-16. With other types of compression-amplification curves, less emphasis is given to the lower level echoes and even the specular echoes may be preferentially amplified (Fig. 1-17). Because of the considerations referred to above, such pre-signal processing to date has not found very wide use. However, there may be times, as for example in the demonstration of metastatic disease, when the contour of the organ needs to be preferentially stressed, and then one of these alternative compression amplification curves would be advantageous.

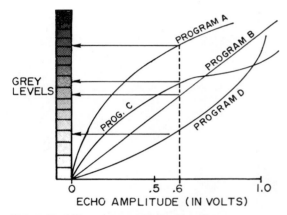

FIG. 1-16. Different types of compression amplification curves which can be employed in pre-signal processing. Program A accentuates the low level echoes and compresses the larger ones, so that an input of 0.6 volts is toward the maximum display intensity. Program B shows linear amplification in which all echoes are equally amplified. Program C shows a sigmoid curve accentuating some low level and some high level echoes with compression of the intermediate echoes. Program D accentuates the higher level echoes (Courtesy of the Picker Corporation).

DISPLAY SYSTEMS

Cathode Ray Tubes (CRT) are a special type of vacuum tube similar to that present in televisions. It produces a narrow beam of electrons which are accelerated towards the anode on the front of the tube (Fig. 1-18). This surface of the tube contains the phosphor layer which glows when an electron beam hits it.

It is now easy to appreciate how a large echo can be modulated into a bright spot. A large echo hitting the transducer causes a large potential difference. This signal is further amplified and processed and eventually fed into the electron gun. A large electrical signal produces more electrons from the electron gun, and this in turn produces a brighter spot on the CRT face. This brightness modulation is known as the Z-axis.

The position of the spot on the CRT face depends on the X-Y coordinates and these relate to the position of the transducer as sensed by the potentiometers in the joints of the scanning arm. Potentials from these position-sensing devices are fed into vertical and horizontal deflection plates within the vacuum tube, which deflect the electron beam correspondingly.

One problem with the CRT is the possibility of excessive intensity. If excessive electrons hit the phosphor, this activity spreads to the surrounding area so that the small echo becomes diffused over a larger area. This results in "blooming" and loss of resolution. Different types of phosphor glow for varying periods of time, that is, they have a different persistence. If there is only transient luminance of the phosphor, some other storage method must be used. One possibility is to expose the transient illumination of the CRT to film for the entire scanning period. This is called the "open shutter technique," and was widely used before the development of scan converters. It resulted in very high quality gray-scale hard copy. Storage phosphor tubes exist, that is, the luminescence can be retained on the face of the CRT and photographed. These photographs tend to result in very poor image quality because of the poor gray-scale characteristics of most phosphors.

A CRT had disadvantages, however. Instability was pronounced with both thermal and aging drift; the signal was not in video format and was therefore not compatible with

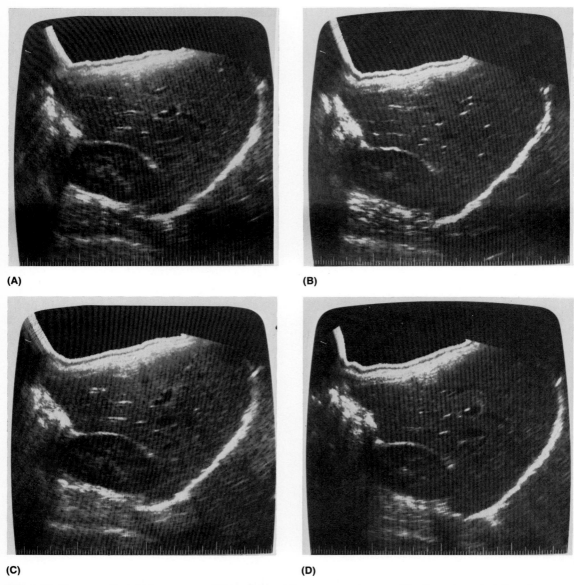

(A)   **(B)**

(C)   **(D)**

FIG. 1-17. The same liver-kidney scans utilizing each of the compression amplification characteristics shown in Figure 16. Note that there is much better parenchymal characterization in A than in D because of the selective amplification of the low level echoes.

TV recorders or video tapes. Considerable skill was also required to obtain a scan without overwriting the same area many times. Such overwriting led to excessive luminance and "blooming" of the phosphor. Because of these difficulties, the analog scan converter was introduced in 1974.

Analog Scan Converters are memory tubes which essentially contain an electron gun which can serve alternatively for writing, reading and erasing. The target for the electron gun consists of a silicon-silicon oxide sandwich about one inch in diameter divided into a matrix of elements around 10 microns

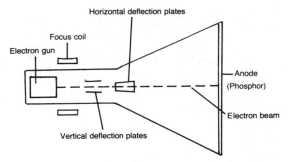

FIG. 1-18. Schema of the cathode ray tube (CRT). Electrons are produced by an electron gun and accelerated towards the phosphor face of the tube. When hit by an electron beam, the phosphor emits light. The beam is directed by horizontal and vertical deflection plates to the X-Y coordinates from the position sensing devices on the scanning arm.

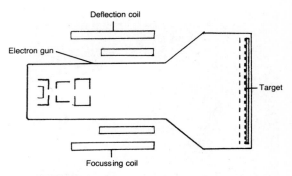

FIG. 1-19. Schema of analog scan converter. The target consists of a silicon-silicon oxide wafer about 25 mm in diameter. Deflection and focusing coils are situated external to the tube.

square. This is shown schematically in Figure 1-19. Again, the X-Y coordinates are controlled by deflection coils external to the tube.

The advantages of an analog scan converter are many. The images are in video format and therefore can be reproduced on inexpensive television monitors. A character generator can be used to add the patient's ID number, date, institution and type of ex-

amination. The image can easily be processed using analog methods such as color coding. Overwriting does not occur, since, if an area is rescanned, the final image replaces the previous one, rather than being added on top of it. There is also a facility to magnify the size of the image or a small part of it by a "zoom" mechanism.

The analog scan converter does have some disadvantages in that there is continuous switching from the reading to writing modes which results in bars over the images at a rate

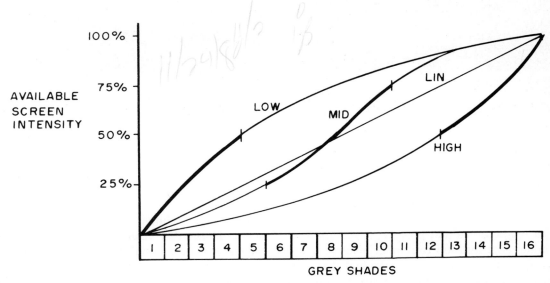

FIG. 1-20. Post-signal processing. This is achieved by a redistribution of gray-scale levels on the display to data in the memory. Note that this data has already been subjected to compression amplification. However, the data can be reallocated to emphasize the low, mid or high level echoes, or a linear display can be given (Courtesy of the Picker Corporation).

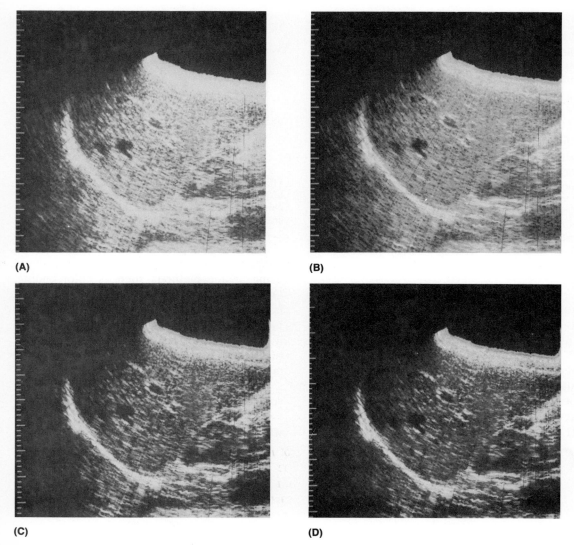

FIG. 1-21. Post-signal processing. **(A)** Accentuation of weak echoes; **(B)** Sigmoidal curve; **(C)** Linear processing; **(D)** Accentuation of strong echoes.

of 10 times for each frame. Another definite disadvantage is that of instability. There is a gradual drift of focus and gray-scale qualities with temperature and time. This results in a gradual deterioration to almost bistable quality. The drift tends to be so gradual that it is often not noticed by the sonographer or ultrasonologist until it has resulted in severe compromise of clinical accuracy. This instability is inherent in the use of a tube. One further prob-

lem with the use of an analog scan converter is the writing speed. Using an analog scan converter, it takes almost 5 seconds to complete a scan. Thus, the scan converter decreases scanning speed. It therefore has no potential for real-time imaging. Both stability and writing speed have been greatly improved by the introduction of digital scan converters.

Digital Scan Converters employ digital memory and circuitry to convert echo signals into an image in TV video format. The cost of large scale digital memory has decreased so much in recent years that this is now a practical, and indeed desirable, alternative to analog scan converters. A digital memory is a solid state, semiconductor device; there is no electron beam to focus or drift in a digital memory; therefore the system, unlike the vacuum storage devices, is completely stable. Problems of focusing, thermal and aging drift no longer occur. The limitation of writing speed also no longer exists since the digital scan converter is capable of reading and writing at the same time. Flicker-free scanning is produced and the system is suitable for real-time imaging. This high-speed writing also allows one to scan on survey mode, in which new information is written over and erases previous information.

Since the information is in digital format, it may be manipulated by the operator during signal processing between the transducer and the memory. This is known as pre-signal processing. It has been seen that this is essentially a change in the compression amplification characteristics of the machine and that any number of different programs can be fed into the system. Further operator manipulation of the data can be carried out between the memory and the display; this is called post-signal processing.

Post-signal Processing is the further manipulation of data to optimize the pathological features of scans. The clinical utility of this procedure is still being assessed. The facility is shown schematically in Figure 1-20. When the data are in the digital memory, there can be a reallocation of gray-scale levels in the display, according to one of the fixed programs available at the touch of a button. The programs available on commercially produced machines include linear, mid-, low-, and high-level echo emphasis. The resulting displays are seen in Figure 1-21A – D.

CONCLUSION

Although the basic physics involved in ultrasound instrumentation has existed for half a century, there have been remarkable improvements in the past 5 years which have resulted first, in gray-scale imaging, and then in increasingly improved resolution. Improvements in transducer design during the past two years have produced a dramatic increase in sensitivity while the introduction of digital scan converters has given a stability hitherto unknown for ultrasound instrumentation. With the data in digital format the entire field of image enhancement and data manipulation becomes a reality, so that the next stage is to employ proven techniques of image enhancement and follow this with the extraction of quantitative information.

2

Real-Time Instrumentation, Automated Imaging, Pulse Doppler Devices

KENNETH J. W. TAYLOR

INTRODUCTION

Real-time is a phrase borrowed from computer jargon. It refers to the dynamic presentation of sequential images, at frame rates of up to 60 per second. This results in a movie of structures as they change position with time. Real-time imaging has two important applications: first, there is the ability to image the movements of fast moving structures such as heart valves; secondly, and equally important, it provides a means for producing automated imaging which is largely independent of the manual skill of the sonographer or ultrasonologist. Since the acquisition of high quality *B-Scans* is presently a major limitation on the development of the entire modality, the ability to produce scans mechanically or electronically has important implications for the future growth of ultrasound usage.

From the consideration of basic physics in the preceeding chapter, it will be recalled that a B-scan is a tomogram which is generated by the movement of the transducer in a single plane across the structure being scanned. Hitherto, we have considered only equipment in which the transducer is moved by hand. In real-time or automated instrumentation, the ultrasound beam is moved in space either mechanically or electronically. A B-mode tomogram can be made either as a sector scan (Fig. 2-1A), a linear scan (Fig. 2-1B) or a combination of both these (Fig. 2-1C). In manual scanning techniques, any of these three types of single-sweep scans can be used, and the combination of a sector scan at either end of a linear scan allows a large volume of anatomy to be shown on the screen, which aids in orientation. To date, automated scanning equipment has been limited either to sector or linear scans, and these will be considered separately. Figure 2-2 shows a schema

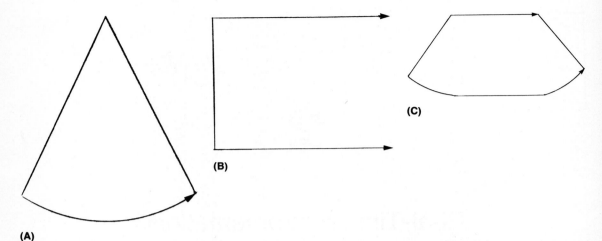

Fig. 2-1. Single pass scanning technique. (A) Single sector scan. (B) Linear scan. (C) Combination of linear and sector scan.

of the way in which we divide most of the real-time, automated ultrasound equipment currently available. Finally, we will consider annular arrays and various multiplex scanners with which the sonographer should be familiar.

Mechanical Linear Scanners

In a mechanical-linear scanner, a single transducer is moved backwards and forwards at high speed. (Fig. 2-3A). Although there are some mechanical disadvantages in such a system, the use of a single transducer element produces a good beam profile, so that the quality of imaging can be good to excellent. The resulting scans from one such mechanical

linear "small parts" scanner are shown in Figures 2-3A–C. This scanner functions at a frequency of 10 MHz and produces outstanding resolution.

Electronic Linear Arrays

Linear arrays have been very successfully utilized, particularly in obstetrics, for the past 5 years. The transducer for a linear array consists of a block of 64 transducers arranged like piano keys, with electrical isolation between each transducer, the entire array measuring approximately 10 cm in length. Obviously, the width of each transducer element must be small. This is a severe disadvantage

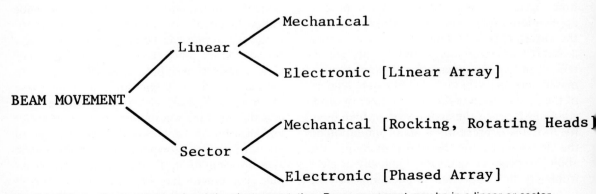

Fig. 2-2. Schema to show types of real-time instrumentation. Beam movement may be in a linear or sector format. Both linear and sector movements of the beam can be produced by mechanical or electronic means.

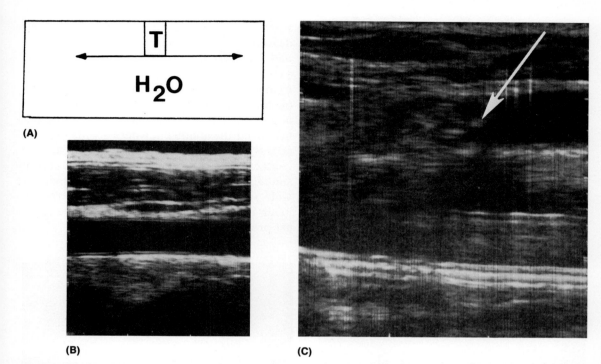

Fig. 2-3. **(A)** Schema to show a mechanical linear scanner in which the transducer in a water bath is moved rapidly to and fro. **(B)** Scan of carotid artery in normal patient, using a linear scanner shown schematically **(A)**. **(C)** Carotid artery stenosis. The site of the obstruction is arrowed.

since, when the transducer size is of the same order as the wave length, a widely divergent ultrasound beam is produced. This problem is solved by activating the transducers in a box of four at a time. Thus, transducers one to four send the first pulse, two to five the second, three to six the third and so on, until 63 scan lines are present. This results in a tomogram which is the length of the transducer and can be 25 cm deep. The entire process can be repeated up to 30 times per second, thereby producing real-time scanning.

For several years the quality obtainable by linear arrays was such that their use was limited to obstetrics. However, increasingly sophisticated instrumentation is now available for scanning the abdomen. With a price range of between \$20,000 and \$34,000, these represent some of the cheapest types of ultrasound instrumentation. This equipment is light and is used at this institution for all portable work.

One disadvantage of the linear array system is that the beam is emitted from a long straight face resulting in poor contact with curved body contours. Since the viewing field is a rectangle, any intercostal sector scans which may be required for scanning the liver or biliary tree cannot be performed (see pp. 102, 116). Another major disadvantage of the system is relatively poor lateral resolution, although gradual improvements are being made. Obviously, if there are only 63 lines in 10 cm, the line density is limited. The number of lines can be doubled electronically to produce more acceptable images without actually improving the resolution. The resolution in the axial plane, however, is good (around 1 mm) since this depends on the pulse length.

More sophisticated linear arrays are now becoming available. These function at 3.5 MHz and 5 MHz with improved lateral resolution. Some of these arrays now have either optical (a lens on the front surface), or even electronic focusing, which will be considered later. A single frame from a linear array is

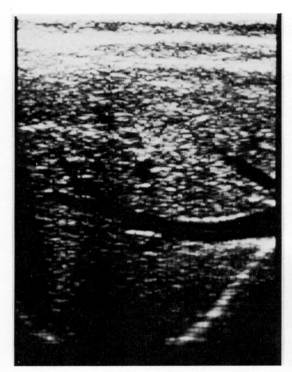

Fig. 2-4. Single frame from a linear array showing excellent resolution of the liver (Courtesy of Narco Air Shields).

which can be varied from 15 degrees to 60 degrees, at a frame rate of up to 60 per second. The resolution of stopped frames can be excellent (Fig. 2-5). The scan is obviously triangular with its apex at the transducer face on the abdominal wall. Such a configuration is particularly advantageous for scanning the heart and the abdomen, where a wide internal access can be obtained with minimal surface contact. Such a scanner is obviously poorly suited to obstetrical scanning where there is wide surface access. Linear arrays provide a much more complete scan in all but the earliest pregnancies.

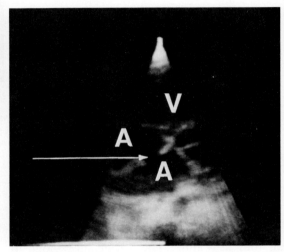

Fig. 2-5. Mechanical sector scan of the heart, scanned from the apex. The ventricles (V) and atria (A) are well displayed. A small septal defect (arrowed) is present (Courtesy of Dr. C. Jaffe).

shown in Figure 2-4. It should be noted that with all real-time instrumentation the apparent resolution is better when viewed dynamically than when presented as a single still frame, or "spot film." The eye integrates a number of frames over a period of time, and this substantially improves the data density. At the same time, the extra information or signal received improves the signal-to-noise ratio so that any electronic noise becomes less noticable. The result of these perceptual changes is a marked improvement of the dynamic image over the spot frame taken as hard copy.

Mechanical Sector Scanners (Rockers, Rotating Transducers)

Simple mechanical sector scanners have been outstandingly successful in imaging the heart, especially in children. The single transducer element is rocked mechanically in a sector

It is important to comprehend the limitations imposed on all real-time systems because of the velocity of sound in tissue. With the sector scanners, it is important to recognize how one can compromise between frame rate and angle of view. The first compromise to consider is that between the number of pulses per second (prf) and the depth of penetration.

It must be recalled that the speed of sound in tissue is approximately 1500 m/s or 150 cm/ms. Thus, in 1 ms a sound beam can traverse 75 cm of tissue and return to the transducer. It should also be recalled that in manual ultrasound systems, 1 millisecond is the time interval between each sequential pulse. Since we never need to go any deeper than 25 cm of tissue, we could increase the number of pulses up to approximately 3000 per second. In the development of real-time imaging, the more scan lines that can be generated in a second, the greater the line density, and the better the resolution (or more frames) produced. It should now be appreciated that if one wants to image to the depth of 25 cm, the maximum number of pulses that can be employed is 3000. Any attempt to use a higher prf results in the echoes from one pulse being superimposed on those from the next pulse. Equally, if one only needs to image 5 cm into the body, as may be true with a newborn, a prf which is five times as high, with improved data density, can be used. Hitherto, the operator has not been provided with such control over the prf, but this is one way in which the rate of acquisition of data could be improved.

Accepting that we have a fixed prf of 3000 pulses per second in a mechanical sector scanner, we have a choice of the way in which we divide these in time and space. If we wish to image a very rapidly moving structure, then we may need 60 frames per second. Since there are 3,000 pulses per second, each scan

has only 50 lines. If we have only 50 lines of data for a very wide angle scan, there is wide separation between the lines and poor resolution (Figs. 2-6A and B). If, however, we can cone our area of interest down to a very small angle, then the data density and the resolution are greatly improved (Fig. 2-6C). When an image moves slowly in time, a low frame rate is adequate, perhaps 15 frames per second. With a prf of 3000, each frame now has 200 lines, so that we can afford the luxury of a wider scan angle without loss of resolution from inadequate scan lines.

A further variation on mechanical sector scanners involves the use of two or more rotating transducers. A rotating transducer surmounts the mechanical problems of discomfort produced by the constant oscillation of the rocking transducer on the skin. The rotating transducers are housed within a head which rotates smoothly just off the surface of the skin. Each transducer, in turn, is used to image a quadrant of interest.

Electronic Sector Scanners (Phased Arrays)

Phased arrays include annular arrays as well as sector scanners, so this type of equipment should be referred to as electronic sector

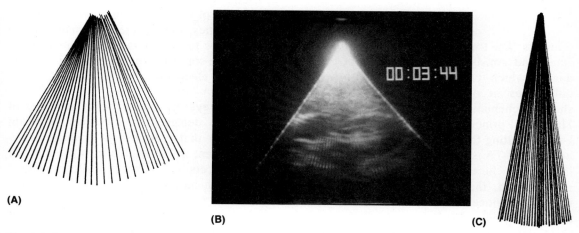

(A)

(B)

(C)

Fig. 2-6. Schema of sector scan to show the effect of data density. **(A)** In fast scanning, a limited number of lines are present, so that a wide sector angle gives definite separation between lines. **(B)** Sector scan showing separation between the individual data lines due to fast wide angle scanning. **(C)** Schema to show how narrowing the angle of view increases the data density.

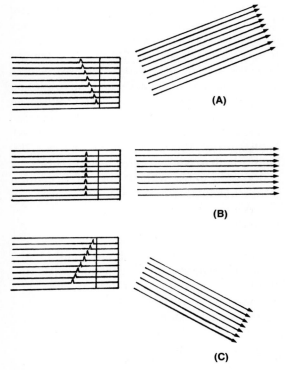

(A)

(B)

(C)

Fig. 2-7. **(A)** Sequential delay in the excitation of each transducer in an array results in the ultrasound beam leaving the transducer face at an angle, according to Huygen's principle. **(B)** Excitation of all transducers simultaneously results in a beam leaving perpendicular to the transducer face. **(C)** Excitation of the transducers with a different delay pattern produces further deviation of the ultrasound beam. Using delays sequentially, an electronic sector scan can be performed.

scanners. The transducers are highly sophisticated and consist of a small block of transducers which can be activated with slight differences in time between each. This is shown schematically in Figure 2-7A. By Huygen's principle (p. 2) the ultrasound beam resulting from transducers activated as in Figure 2-7A is emitted at an angle from the face. Since the whole pulse lasts less than a microsecond, the delay between the activation of transducers is minute and is measured in nanoseconds (10^{-9} seconds). Obviously this delay in activation must be infinitely variable. When all the transducers are activated together, the beam passes parallel to the transducer (Fig. 2-7B), while sequential delay in

the opposite direction causes the beam to be deviated downwards (Fig. 2-7C). This results in electronic steering of the beam which has been successfully applied to imaging the heart. This principle has not found great application in imaging the abdomen to date, partly because of the expense (approximately $100,000), but also because of the relatively poor resolution compared to a simple single-element transducer. These sophisticated systems have quite marked side lobes or "grating" lobes which are regions of appreciable ultrasound energy located on either side of the beam axis. A large reflection from the grating lobes will be interpreted as a reflector on the main axis of the beam and will lead to considerable artifacts. One attraction of these systems is the possibility of focusing the beam by suitable excitation of the transducers (Fig. 2-8).

Electronic arrays are sophisticated devices requiring large scale computers for successful switching of the transducer elements. This computerized control, and the delay lines necessary to produce the electronic delay for transducer activation, is responsible for the great expense of these systems. The possibility of electronic beam steering and focusing has caused tremendous excitement in the past few years, but there is increasing acknowledgment of the difficulties of adequate suppression of side lobes, as well as the cost of the instrumentation. In view of the difficulties, development of instrumentation appears to be moving predominantly towards more sophisticated mechanical systems rather than electronic arrays.

Annular Arrays An annular array is a nest of transducers designed to improve the beam profile over that produced by a single transducer element. In an annular array, a number of transducers are concentrically arranged. Each transducer focuses at a different distance so that by the use of all transducers, a thin-beam profile should be obtained. Because of the number of transducers involved, the transducer head tends to be large, and skin contact becomes more difficult. In practice, from the clinical evaluations that have been carried

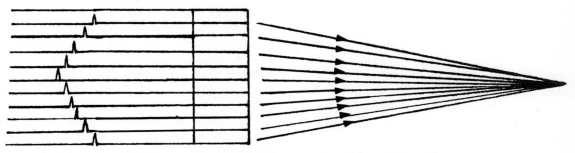

Fig. 2-8. Schema of phased array to show how excitation of the central transducers can lead to a focused beam. The focusing characteristics are infinitely variable with the various delays that can be employed.

out, the improvement in resolution for clinical scanning appears to be rather marginal. The future of annular arrays at present appears uncertain, and cost effectiveness over a focused single element is unproven.

Specific Multiplex Mechanical Scanners We will now consider a number of mechanical scanners which have recently appeared on the market. These are more complex than the simple mechanical systems considered so far.

The Octoson is a mechanical, and hence automatic, ultrasound imaging system devised by George Kossoff in Sydney, Australia. For more than 5 years, this machine has been producing some of the most elegant scans. The Octoson was the prototype of the "water path" scanners, the design of which is based on solid physical principles. We have already considered the complexity of the ultrasound intensity profile close to the transducer face, compared to the more even field further from the transducer (pp. 13–14). When a transducer is in contact with the skin, the first 4-5 cm of the imaged tissue lies before the region of focus in most clinically used transducers. From the point of view of physics, it is therefore logical to have the transducer some distance away from the skin in a water bath so that the tissue to be imaged lies in the focal zone of the transducer. Unfortunately, there are complications with such an approach since reverberations occur, which will be considered in the next chapter. The result of reverberation is the necessity for scanning away from the skin the same distance as the depth to which one wishes to image. Thus, since

we frequently image to 20 cm, the transducer must be at least 20 cm from the skin.

In the Octoson system, eight transducers are arranged in a semicircle in a water bath and are moved mechanically through an arc. The patient lies face down on a membrane

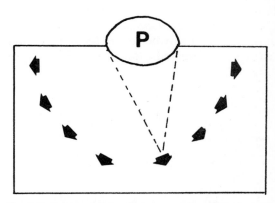

Fig. 2-9. Schema of the Octoson system (mechanical sector scanner). Eight transducers are moved through a sector motion to produce a compounded scan. P is the patient.

surface of the water bath (Fig. 2-9). As each transducer moves through an arc, a compounded scan is made. The major advantages of this system are that it produces superb resolution, it is entirely automatic and it is possible to put patients through quickly, perhaps up to 50 per day. The disadvantages of the system are that it is extremely expensive when compared to other ultrasound instrumentation; the water bath makes it a very large piece of equipment; it suffers the disadvantages of compound scanning, which include degradation of axial resolution and some multiple registrations of single reflectors due to incorrect assumption of velocity. The real-time potential is relatively low since the addition of a water path decreases the number of pulses that can be used compared to direct contact, real-time machines or those with a more limited water path, as described below.

The Annular array system with water path is essentially a mechanical sector scanner which incorporates the use of an annular array and a moving mirror in a water bath. A schema of such an instrument is shown in Figure 2-10A, and the resulting scan in Figure 2-10B. This system uses the water path principle, and a sector scan is produced by mechanically rocking the mirror from which the beam is reflected. This system has the following advantages: good resolution, although one should compare this objectively to the resolution obtained by single-element transducers, good imaging because the water path enables the target to be in the focal zone, and entirely automated imaging. The disad-

vantages of the system are that there is a large scanning head and a large area of contact is required (this is a disadvantage when compared to the sector scanning devices in contact with the skin, where minimal surface contact can be used to provide maximum display of internal anatomy) and that the real-time potential is limited, again because of the low pulse rate resulting from the amount of time which the beam takes to traverse the water path as well as the tissue. This instrument, however, is a further highly ingenious attempt to produce automated scanning with resolution of the manual B-scanner. It is obvious that all these automated scanners are most appropriate in hospitals with inadequate numbers of highly trained sonographers or ultrasonologists to obtain manual scans.

The Hand Held Mechanical Scanner With Water Path is a further innovative approach which attempts to reduce the size of the scanning head to a hand-held device, while retaining the advantages of a water path. The long water path utilized in other systems is necessitated by the mismatch be-

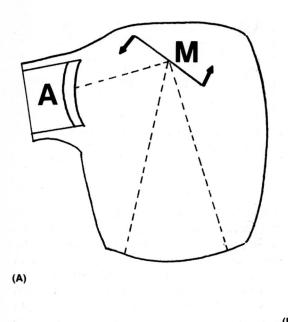

(A)

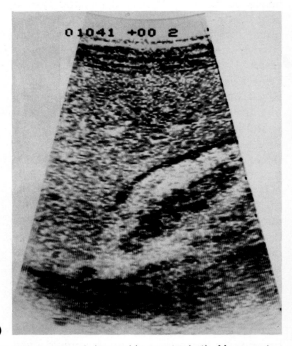

(B)

Fig. 2-10. **(A)** Schema to show annular array (mechanical sector scanner), housed in a water bath. Movement of the beam is produced by mechanically moving the mirror. **(B)** Scan through the liver and right kidney, using the annular array shown schematically in Figure 2-11A.

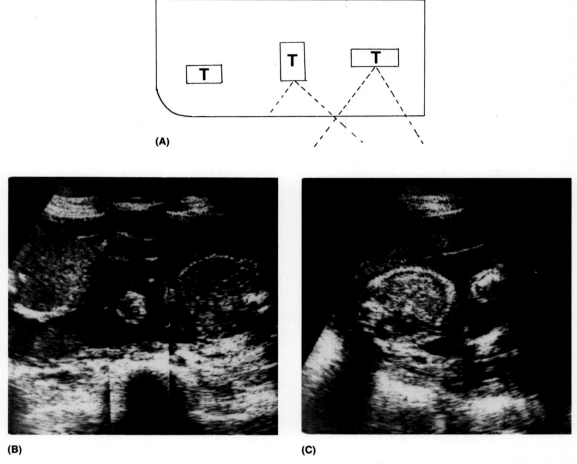

Fig. 2-11 **(A)** Mechanical sector scanner. Schema to show three transducers in a water bath with production of a compounded scan. Careful coupling between the fluid and the transducer overcomes the problems of reverberation. **(B, C)** Obstetrical scans showing resolution of the scanner described in Figure 11A.

tween the transducer and the fluid path, which results in reverberation. This problem was solved by using a fluid which was well matched with the transducer, thereby preventing reverberation. With this system, the transducer can be only 3 cm from the skin surface but can move freely in a linear or sector scan within its fluid bath. A schema of this equipment is shown in Figure 2-11A and resulting scans in Figures 2-11B & C. This system has not undergone adequate clinical evaluation at this point, to permit enumeration of advantages and disadvantages.

Rotating Transducers With Pulsed Doppler Device. This system is one of the fore-runners of a group of mechanical scanners utilizing rotating transducers. This results in high quality automatic imaging and relatively low cost. In addition, a pulsed Doppler facility is available.

Continuous Wave Doppler. The *Doppler principle* refers to a change in frequency when sound or ultrasound is emitted from a moving source. The simplest example is that of a siren, which when coming towards the listener has a rising frequency. As the siren goes away from the listener, the frequency appears to decrease. This principle can be appreciated best by considering the schema shown in Figures 2-12 A–C. Figure 2-12 A

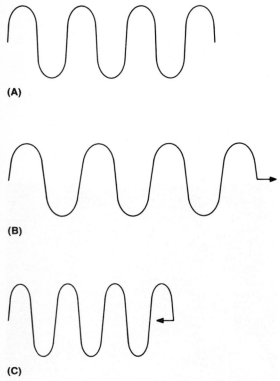

(A)

(B)

(C)

Fig. 2-12. Doppler principle. **(A)** Sine wave representing sound wave of a given frequency. **(B)** If the source of the sine wave is moving away from the receiver, the wavelength is increased and the frequency is lowered. **(C)** If the sound source is moving towards the receiver, the wavelength is shorter and the frequency is increased.

shows a sine wave representing a sound wave of a given frequency. If the source of that sound was moving while the sound was being emitted, the same number of waves would be emitted, but the pulse length would be increased by movement of the source, the result being that the sine wave would be extended like a spring (Fig. 2-12B). An increase of wavelength results in a lower frequency. This change in frequency is known as the Doppler shift. When a source of sound is coming towards the observer, the reverse occurs, that is, the sine wave is compressed, the wavelength shortened and the frequency increased (Fig. 2-12C).

In Doppler ultrasound techniques, a

sound wave is bounced off moving structures, most frequently red blood cells, which therefore act as if they were moving sources of ultrasound. If the red cell is moving in the plane of the ultrasound beam, then the Doppler shift (that is the increase in frequency as the red cell comes towards the transducer) is directly proportional to the velocity of the red cell. Conversely, if the red cell is moving away from the transducer in the plane of the ultrasound beam, the fall in frequency (Doppler shift) is again directly proportional to the velocity of the moving red cell. Thus, the Doppler shift can tell us not only the velocity of red cell movement but also its direction. Most frequently the plane of the red cell motion will not coincide with the plane of the ultrasound beam, and if absolute velocity needs to be calculated, allowance must be made for the angle between the sound beam and the red cell movement. It may be difficult or impossible to assess this angle, so that absolute velocity may be difficult to calculate. However, the important aspects of Doppler use in clinical practice are the ability to determine the presence and direction of flow.

Pulse Doppler Devices So far we have considered a continuous Doppler device, i.e., a continuous Doppler beam is emitted from the transducer face. Such a beam may traverse many blood vessels, for example the portal vein and inferior vena cava, as well as many smaller hepatic or gastric veins. With such a device we cannot pinpoint the site of the Doppler shift in relation to its depth from the transducer face. We are able to do this by combining the Doppler device with a B-scan. The distance from the transducer face at which the Doppler shift was measured is noted, and this will clarify whether the signal is from the portal vein or the inferior vena cava, for example. Spatial discrimination is provided by the use of the pulse Doppler principle. A short envelope of ultrasound waves is emitted from the transducer, and then the position of a gate is adjusted to accept only those echoes emanating from a given distance from the transducer. This gate can be adjusted to any chosen position from inspection of the B-scan, which is obtained simultaneously. Such a piece of equipment has many uses which have been clinically evaluated at this institution. In particular, the ability to detect a Doppler shift and normal venous flow excludes venous thrombosis. The ability to differentiate between arterial and venous structures, vascular malformations and aneurysms is extremely valuable, particularly when the normal anatomy is distorted by extensive pathology. This equipment has also been used to differentiate bile ducts from portal vein radicles, to detect turbulence associated with atrial septal defects, as well as assessing flow in veins.

CONCLUSION

The field of ultrasonic instrumentation is changing extremely rapidly. Nevertheless, the basic principles considered here should allow the objective assessment of new equipment as it becomes available. In the abdomen, there is some value in being able to view dynamic anatomy. But a major advantage of real-time systems is the ability to use automated scanning. We have now arrived at a stage in which

the quality of the B-scan can be almost independent of the skill of the operator. Ultrasound "fluoroscopy" is now a reality. However, unlike X-ray fluoroscopy, freedom from harmful bioeffects allows us to leave the scanning procedure in the hands of the sonographer who has been trained to recognize pathology and document its presence for the physician.

SUGGESTED READING

Garrett WJ, Kossoff G, Carpenter DA: The Octoson in use. In: Ultrasound in Medicine, Vol. II, ed. White D, Brown R. New York, Plenum Press, 1976.

Griffith JM, Henry WL: A sector scanner for real time two-dimensional echocardiography. Circulation 49: 1147, 1974.

Green PS, Taenzer JC, Ramsey JF, et al: A real time ultrasound imaging system for cardio-arteriography. Ultrasound Med Biol 3:129, 1977.

Holm HH, Kristensen JK, Petersen JF, Hancke S, Northeved A: A new mechanical real time ultrasonic scanner. Ultrasound Med Biol 2:19, 1975.

Shirley IM, Blackwell RJ, Cusick G. Farman DJ, Vicary FR: A Users Guide to Diagnostic Ultrasound. Baltimore, Pitman Medical, 1978.

Taylor KJW, Atkinson P, deGraaff CS, et al: Clinical evaluation of pulse-doppler device linked to gray scale B-scan equipment. Radiology 129:745-749, 1978.

3

Artifacts and Pitfalls

KENNETH J. W. TAYLOR

INTRODUCTION

After reading this chapter the reader may be bewildered about whether one can ever obtain reliable clinical information without being misled by artifacts. That is precisely the reason this chapter is so important for the student sonographer and the ultrasonologist. All of us have made errors in diagnosis because artifacts were not appreciated or because of physical effects we did not understand. Therefore, we will consider the artifacts and pitfalls which commonly occur and suggest the possible physical mechanisms which cause them.

REVERBERATION

Reverberations are due to the relatively large impedance mismatch between tissues and the transducer face. When an echo returns from these tissues, an appreciable proportion of it may be reflected back into the tissues instead of passing into the transducer. This gives rise to the possibility that an ultrasound beam may have multiple paths between the transducer face and a large reflector within tissues before it is finally received back into the tranduser. Reverberations normally occur between the transducer face and a large reflector such as the rectus sheath or the posterior wall of the bladder. These reverberations are particularly noticeable in obese patients. When an echo is received from an interface, the position of that interface is correctly located at the appropriate distance from the transducer by calculating the time of flight and velocity of sound in tissue. However, if part of that energy is reflected back into the tissues and bounces off the same reflector again before being received by the transducer, the time taken for this path is twice that of the first echo, and the reflector

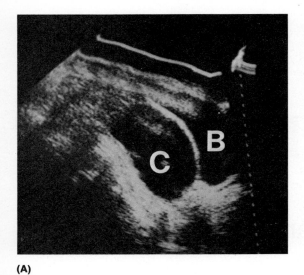

(A)

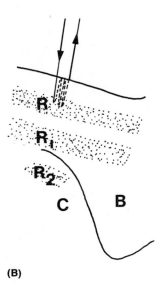

(B)

Fig. 3-1 **(A)** Reverberation artifact. A pelvic scan in the parasagittal plane showing a dilated urinary bladder (B), and a fluid collection (C) posterior to the bladder. Notice there are multiple artifacts in both cystic collections shown schematically in Figure 3-1B. **(B)** Schema to show the production of reverberation artifacts. The ultrasound beam reverberates between the transducer face and a reflector such as the rectus sheath (R). When a single reverberation occurs, the returning echo has taken twice the amount of time to travel from the skin to the reflector, so that the first reverberation is placed in the position indicated by R_1. Further reverberations may occur by a similar mechanism indicated by R_2. Each reverberation is of lower amplitude than the preceding one, since only a fraction of the energy is reflected at the transducer face.

is imaged again at twice the distance between the transducer and the first reflector (Figs. 3-1A and B). If a second reverberation occurs, a further interface is seen. Thus, reverberations are seen as repetitions of a reflector, equidistant from each other and the same distance as the transducer to the first reflector. Figure 3-1A shows an actual pelvic scan and this mechanism is shown schematically in Figure 3-1B. Reverberations are commonly seen in superficial cystic collections, such as amniotic fluid, the gallbladder or urinary bladder. This results in a series of echoes on the proximal surface of the cystic collection which simulate the presence of interfaces within it. The novice may be misled into believing that there is solid material in the wall of the bladder or that echoes represent an anterior placenta. With experience, reverberations are immediately recognized and excluded as artifacts. Each reverberation is noted to be less than the preceding one because only a fraction of the energy is reflected from the transducer face each time, and the

fractions become ever smaller.

Occurence of reverberations is a particular problem common in attempting to utilize the water path principle. Because of the complexity of the ultrasound field and the beam widths adjacent to the transducer, the object to be imaged should be ideally in the focal zone of the transducer. For superficial organs such as the thyroid, this is most easily achieved by the use of a water path. Figure 3-2A shows the reverberation which occurs as the result of this. To avoid destroying image quality a reverberation must be placed away from the area of interest, and this is achieved by standing off in a water bath at a greater distance than the depth to which one wishes to image. Thus, the reverberations are placed posterior to the area of interest. (Fig. 3-2B).

It is because of this problem with reverberation in a water path that the ultrasound systems using this approach have had to employ transducers standing 20 cm from the skin surface to image to a distance of 20 cm. The

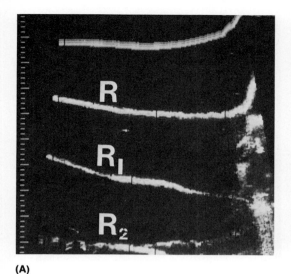

(A)

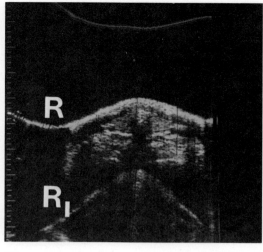

(B)

Fig. 3-2 **(A)** Multiple reverberations (R, R$_1$, R$_2$) are seen from scanning in a water bath. Note that the distance between the reverberations is the same as that between the transducer and the first reflector. **(B)** Water bath scanning of the thyroid. Notice the reverberation (R$_1$) from the skin surface (R). When the transducer stands off from the skin surface, the reverberation can be placed posterior to the area of interest.

recent introduction of much shorter water paths (p. 31) stems from an innovative approach to match the coupling fluid to the transducer so that no appreciable echo formation occurs at the transducer face.

ACOUSTIC SHADOWING

An acoustic shadow is due to a loss of ultrasound energy distal to a reflector. There appear to be a number of mechanisms responsible for this phenomenon, including attenuation, refraction and reflection.

Acoustic Shadowing Due to Attenuation is seen most commonly beyond bone and gallstones. Figure 3-3A shows the very distinct distal shadow due to the high attenuation of the gallstone. Gallstones attenuate sound both by reflection and absorption. Our measurements have indicated that gallstones attenuate around 14 dB, so that the normal TGC which compensates for soft tissue attenuation is inadequate compensation for very high attenuation by gallstones. A similar phenomenon is seen distal to the dense collagen in scar tissue, posterior to air or barium in the

gut, or bone (Fig. 3-3B). Calcification always gives rise to acoustic shadowing providing that the TGC is adjusted appropriately, so that a calcified fibroid will also shadow.

Acoustic Shadowing Due to Refraction It has long been noted that shadows may be seen from the edges of cystic structures. At the edge of a cystic lesion within soft tissue, there is an interface between media of different acoustic velocities. The velocity of sound in water is 1460 m/s and in tissue 1540 m/s. As with a light beam, an ultrasound beam is bent or refracted at this interface. After transmission through the cystic contents, the beam is again refracted at the tissue/cyst interface, so that the beam emerges parallel to the incident beam. This effect is shown in Figure 3-4A, which is a transverse section through an aortic aneurysm. Notice that there are shadows from each side of the aneurysm which can be explained in terms of the refraction shown schematically in Figure 3-4B. Other sites of refractive shadowing include the gallbladder, liver and kidney cysts, and the fetal bladder.

Acoustic Shadowing Due to Reflection is almost invariably seen in obstetrical scanning. The fetus is surrounded by amniotic flu-

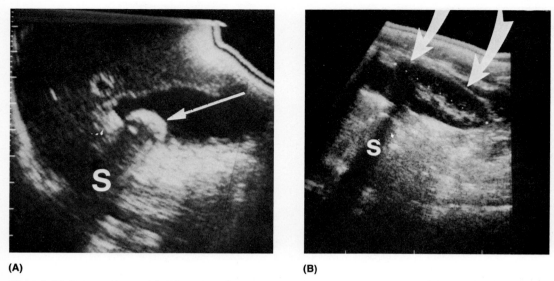

Fig. 3-3 **(A)** B-scan of a gallbladder containing a large gallstone (arrowed). Because of the high attenuation of gallstones, there is an acoustic shadow (S) beyond the stone. **(B)** Longitudinal section through the left kidney (arrowed). There is definite shadowing (S) from rib overlying the kidney.

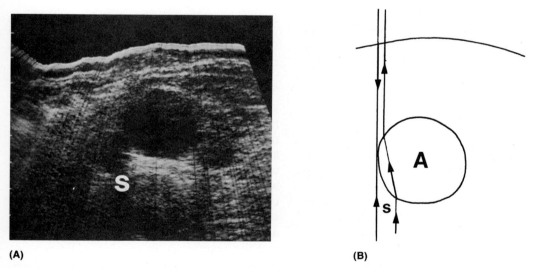

Fig. 3-4 **(A)** Transverse scan through an aortic aneurysm. A definite shadow is seen (S) on each edge of the cystic area. **(B)** Possible mechanism of the shadow formation seen in Fig. 3-4A, based on refraction. The cystic area (A) refracts the beam (shown schematically), leaving a shadow (S) between the direct beam which is not refracted, and the beam which is.

id, and the beam may be reflected at the surface of the fetal body. A well defined acoustic shadow can be seen posterior to the fetal head or the fetal trunk. It was once considered that this was due to attenuation by the skull, but careful examination shows that the shadow is not merely limited to that part of the beam passing through the thickest part of the skull. A more logical explanation has been proposed by Sommer and Filly. They suggest that at the

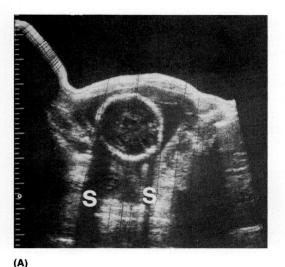

(A)

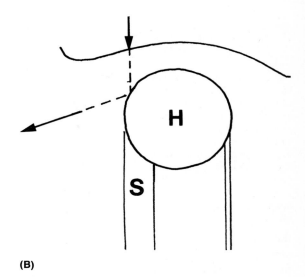

(B)

Fig. 3-5 **(A)** Transverse section to show the fetal head, with definite shadowing (S) behind it. **(B)** Schema to show the possible mechanism for the shadow seen in Figure 3-5A. The fetal head (H) acts as a specular reflector, reflecting the beam and causing the shadow (S).

surface of the fetal body the beam is reflected in a specular manner so that no energy returns to the transducer. Such well marked shadowing is shown in Figure 3-5A and explained schematically in Figure 3-5B.

REVERSE SHADOWING

Reverse shadowing is a phenomenon seen in all cystic lesions when the TGC is set for normal tissue attenuation. Since the attenuation of water is so much lower than that of tissue, if the TGC is set for soft tissue, but the beam traverses water, then the echoes from beyond the cyst are overamplified. Thus, the phenomenon of reverse shadowing is really a result of inappropriate TGC. Elicitation of a reverse shadow remains one of the important criteria for the diagnosis of cysts.

EFFECTS OF BEAM WIDTH

There are important clinical implications from the effect of beam width which have not been adequately considered until recently. Their importance has recently been investigated at this institution. The beam profile of a focused

transducer has already been considered in Chapter 1, (pp. 13–14). It may be recalled that the ultrasound beam is wide as it leaves the transducer and is brought to focus at some distance from the transducer face. Beyond the focal zone the beam diverges. This is shown schematically in Figure 3-6, and has the following important clinical applications.

Nonshadowing Gallstones There have been numerous attempts to correlate the failure of gallstones to shadow with their chemical composition. This merely reflects a lack of appreciation for the basic principles of diagnostic ultrasound. The problem of the lack of shadow is considered further in the chapter on Biliary system (p. 119). One possible mechanism for this phenomenon is that shown schematically in Figure 3-6. Close to the surface of the transducer, the beam width can be 10-15 mm, while in the focal zone it will be reduced to around 3 mm. A 4 mm gallstone represented in the schema completely occludes the beam when placed in the focal zone, and a definite shadow is seen behind it. If, however, the gallstone is adjacent to the transducer face or in the far zone, the beam is not totally occluded so that a shadow is not appreciated. Therefore, since it is important to place small stones in

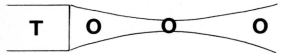

Fig. 3-6. The ultrasound beam emerging from a focused transducer is wide adjacent to the transducer face and is brought into a narrow zone around 9 cm from the transducer. If 'O' represents a gallstone, the beam will be occluded and produce distal shadowing only when the gallstone is in the focal zone of the transducer. If the target 'O' represents a cystic structure, it will only appear completely cystic when it is in the focal zone of the transducer. At distances before and beyond the focal zone, echoes from the surrounding solid tissues will be seen.

the focal zone of the transducer to elicit a shadow, one must be aware of the beam profile of each transducer in clinical use.

Delineation of Small Cystic Areas The successful delineation of small cystic structures is also partially dependent on the beam width, which can be appreciated by considering Figure 3-6. Attention has been drawn to this by Carson. If the object (0) is now considered to be a small cystic lesion, when the small cyst is in the focal zone of the transducer, there is a complete absence of echoes from the cystic area and its nature is recognized. However, if the small cystic lesion is situated in the near or far field, echoes from the surrounding solid tissue are received at the transducer so that the cystic nature of the lesion may not be appreciated. This is analogous to the "partial volume effect," described for CT scanning. This phenomenon is due to a substantial thickness of the X-ray beamwidth. Thus, when the beamwidth encompasses both solid and cystic tissues the X-ray absorption is averaged between the two, and the cystic nature becomes less obvious.

Confusion Between the Contents of Adjacent Viscera Confusion between the contents of adjacent viscera may have very severe clinical implications and is again due to a partial volume effect or beam width consideration. In practice, this confusion is commonly produced by the juxtaposition of the gallbladder, the duodenum and the colon. Material in the duodenum and colon may appear to be within

the lumen of the gallbladder (Fig. 3-7) and the result is the erroneous diagnosis of gallstones and unnecessary surgery. This mistake can be avoided in clinical practice by moving the patient and demonstrating the stones in another part of the gallbladder where there is no chance of the beam also traversing the duodenum or colon.

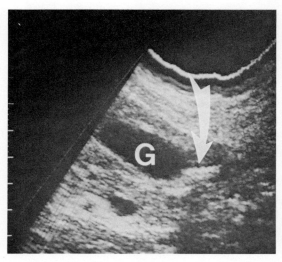

Fig. 3-7. Partial volume effect due to beam width. The gallbladder is seen (G) and a particle (arrowed) in the adjacent colon appears to protrude into the tip of the gallbladder.

Tissue Texture The beam width also has an important implication for the demonstration of true tissue texture. Examination of a scan through a homogeneous organ such as the liver reveals three definite zones (Fig. 3-8). Close to the transducer there is a very fine pattern. Comparison with the beam profile (p. 14) shows that the beam is extremely irregular and complex in this zone. Thus, any single reflector may give a number of echoes from this side or "grating" lobe. The apparent fine tissue architecture seen in this part of the beam is dependent upon the complexity of the beam profile and not representative of the tissue texture itself. In the focal zone of the transducer, the beam width is minimal and maximum echoes are returned from each point reflector. This zone is the zone of true tissue characterization. Finally, in the far zone the echoes become wider, demonstrating the defocusing effect of the beam profile.

Echogenicity of Tissue in the Focal Zone Examination of any clinical B-scan shows that reflectors in the focal zone of the transducer produce larger echoes than those in the near and far zones. (Fig. 3-8) It therefore follows that when echogenicities of various tissues are compared they should be compared at the same distance from the transducer face, and preferably in the focal zone. It has been noted by various authors that retroperitoneal fat appears to be more echogenic than subcutaneous tissue, and it appears probable that this due to beam profile effects. The retroperitoneum lies in the focal zone of most transducers used for clinical practice, while subcutaneous fat tissue lies in the near zone.

lems in obtaining appropriate TGC. Passage of the ultrasound beam through fluid leads to excessive amplification of echoes by the addition of TGC for soft tissues. Thus, echoes from the liver may appear exaggerated due to this technical effect, and simulate cirrhosis. This effect must be differentiated from a cirrhotic liver which is a very common cause for ascites.

A further common artifact seen in ascites is a thickened gallbladder wall (Fig. 3-9). This has been noted by many authors and the precise reasons for it are not apparent. However a large tissue/fluid interface exaggerated by the effects of inappropriate TGC appears to result in a widening of the echo leading to artifactual thickening of the gallbladder wall.

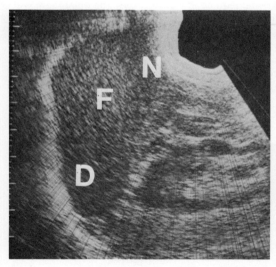

Fig. 3-8. There are three types of texture seen on this scan, and these are related to the focal plane of the transducer. In the near zone (N) there is fine tissue texture. Maximum amplitude of echoes and true liver texture occur in the focal zone (F). In the distal zone (D) the echoes become longer as the lateral resolution deteriorates and the beam becomes defocused and divergent.

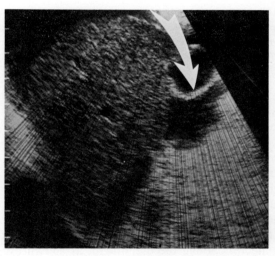

Fig. 3-9. Section through the right lobe of the liver in a patient with extensive ascites, seen as an echo free layer around the liver. Notice that the gallbladder wall (arrowed) appears thick; this thickness does not correlate well with appearances seen at surgery.

EFFECT OF ASCITES

Extensive ascites makes it very difficult to evaluate tissue texture since there are prob-

Echoes Across the Diaphragm

When a routine parasagittal scan through the right upper quadrant is examined, especially at high gain, multiple echoes are seen above the diaphragm, which are clearly artifactual, since this area is occupied by an aerated lung and no part of the ultrasound beam can penetrate it. This is seen in Figure 3-10A, and schema

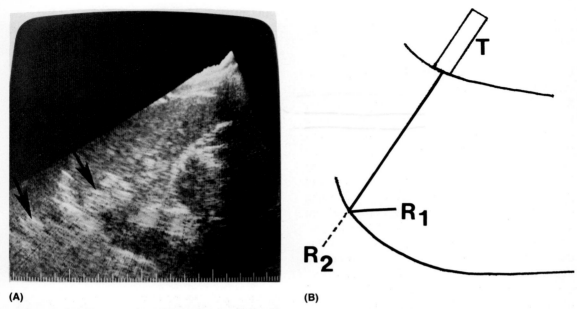

(A)   **(B)**

Figs. 3-10**A** and **B.** Parasagittal section through the liver. Note that there are multiple echoes above the diaphragm which might be partially due to the mechanisms demonstrated in Figure 3-10B. The diaphragm is seen to act as a concave mirror; the mirror image of an echogenic mass (R_1) above the diaphragm (arrowed), is seen below it (R_2, arrowed).

shown in Figure 3-10B suggests the mechanisms for this which were proposed by Cosgrove. It is suggested that the diaphragm acts as a concave mirror for the reflection of the ultrasound beam and echoes from below the diaphragm are reflected off the cavity of the diaphragm before they return to the transducer. During signal processing it is assumed that the beam has returned in a straight line from reflectors above the diaphragm, as shown by the dotted line (Fig. 3-10B). Thus, an infradiaphragmatic reflector (R_1) is projected as a supradiaphragmatic reflector (R_2).

Pseudotumors

A number of abdominal and pelvic masses are seen which may simulate tumors and must be carefully differentiated by the experienced sonographer. Common examples are as follows.

Ligamentum Teres The ligamentum teres is frequently surrounded by varying amounts of fat, especially in males. This gives rise to an echogenic mass in the liver, which can simulate an echogenic metastasis (Fig. 3-11).

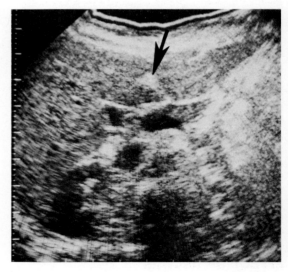

Fig. 3-11. Transverse scan of the upper abdomen. The ligamentum teres (arrowed) appears as an echogenic mass in the liver, but must not be confused with an echogenic metastasis.

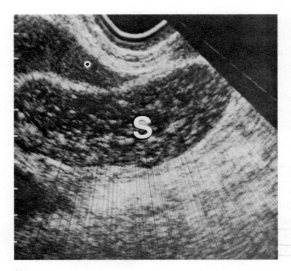

(A)

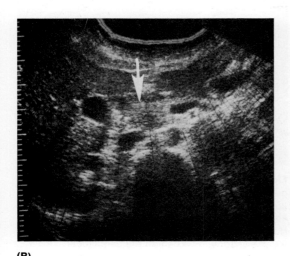

(B)

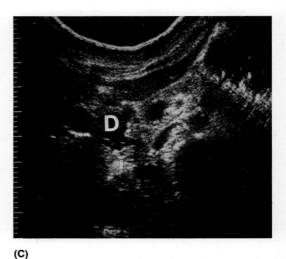

(C)

Fig. 3-12. **(A)** Longitudinal section through the left upper quadrant showing a large mass (S) which contains fine debris. Further investigation reveals that this was merely food in the stomach. **(B)** Transverse section through the upper abdomen. There appears to be a mass in the head of the pancreas (arrowed), but this might be food in the duodenum. **(C)** Ingestion of a quantity of fluid which distends the duodenum (D), shows that the head of the pancreas is normal, and there is no evidence of any tumor.

Upper Abdominal Masses Due to Stomach or Colon Both colon and stomach may simulate pathological upper abdominal masses (Fig. 3: 12A-C). The stomach in particular frequently simulates a pseudocyst of the lesser sac and must be differentiated. Techniques for aiding the recognition of stomach include distention by ingestion of water or carbonated beverage or aspiration if a nasogastric tube is in place. Pseudo tumors due to feces in the colon are most easily differentiated by repeating the examination on the following day.

Pseudotumors in Pelvis Due to Colon and Small Intestinal Contents Pelvic tumors are frequently simulated by small intestinal loops in the Pouch of Douglas or colonic contents. Loops of gut which contain fluid must be differentiated from significant fluid collections due to abscess formation. This is most easily achieved by repetition when gut contents show considerable variation. In patients with inflammatory bowel disease and adhesions, differentiation may be difficult or impossible.

Highly reflective feces in the sigmoid colon simulate the appearance of a dermoid cyst (Fig. 3-13). In some laboratories water enemas are being enthusiastically used to exclude the possibility of colon contents being mistaken for a tumor. In clinical practice, this difference can be successfully achieved by repetition of the examination on the following day, and water enemas have not achieved a wide popularity with our patients or sonographers.

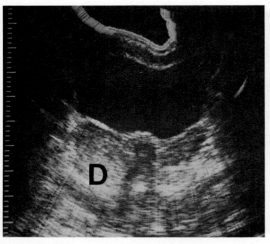

Fig. 3-13. Transverse section through the pelvis, showing a large, highly reflective right adnexal mass (D). These appearances are very highly suggestive of a dermoid cyst. However, at surgery no dermoid cyst was found. The incorrect diagnosis of tumor was made due to visualization of colonic contents.

Scattering From Suspension of Particles Mimicking Solid Consistency

Although ultrasound is capable of differentiating between solid and cystic consistency with an accuracy of approximately 98 percent, occasionally this accuracy will be compromised by the presence of particulate matter within a fluid suspension. Numerous examples

of this are seen in clinical practice and include an organizing hematoma, debris within an abscess or inspissated bile. Any of these fluid collections may appear virtually solid because of the scattering of particulate matter within them. Although liver abscesses are generally sufficiently echo free to be diagnosed correctly as fluid collections, occasionally they may be strongly echogenic and be misdiagnosed as solid lesions. Figure 3-14 shows an obstructed gallbladder which is highly echogenic due to microcrystals contained within.

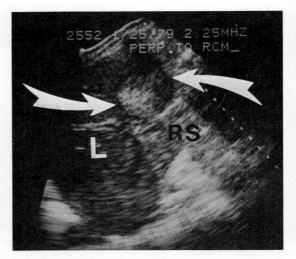

Fig. 3-14. Sector scan through the right upper quadrant showing the liver (L). The gallbladder lumen is arrowed. Notice that it is not echo-free, but contains highly reflective material which is debris. Notice also that the attenuation is low and there is a reverse shadow (RS) behind the gallbladder. These appearances suggest that there is scattering of the beam due to the particles in suspension, but low attenuation.

CONCLUSION

In this chapter we have attempted to describe some of the common artifacts and pitfalls which can confuse and compromise clinical accuracy. Some of the mechanisms are still tentative, and most have been recognized only recently. However, this is probably the most important chapter in this book. Although the literature is filled with reports about the diagnostic success of ultrasound, there are relatively few reports of the common pitfalls which may cause disillusionment with the technique in every day practice by the neophyte. Nothing is more disasterous for our clinical colleagues than to find that results reported enthusiastically in the literature can not be obtained at their own institutions. Those who have been in ultrasound for a long period of time have made all the mistakes resulting from the artifacts and pitfalls discussed, and hopefully by pointing out their errors to others, further confusion can be minimized or prevented.

SUGGESTED READING

Bartrum RJ, Crow HC: Gray-scale Ultrasound: A Manual for Physicians and Technical Personnel, Chapter 5. Philadelphia, W.B. Saunders Co., 1977.

Carson PL, Oughton TV: A modeled study for diagnosis of small anechoic masses with ultrasound. Radiology 122:765, 1977.

Jaffe CC, Taylor KJW: Clinical impact of ultrasonic beam focusing patterns. Radiology 131:469–472, 1979.

Sommer FG, Filly RA, Minton MJ: Acoustic shadowing due to refractive and reflective effects. AJR 132:973–977, 1979.

Taylor KJW, Jacobson P, Jaffe CC: Lack of an acoustic shadow on scans of gallstones: a possible artifact. Radiology 131:463–464, 1979.

4

Establishing an Ultrasound Facility

RALPH WINTERS

A large number of hospitals are currently considering or actually initiating an ultrasound department. Many questions can arise during this process. The solutions to questions involving room size, furnishing, filing space and equipment are often decided by those with limited knowledge of the day-to-day functioning of an ultrasound laboratory. It is the purpose of this chapter to help the sonographer anticipate these questions and to aid in formulating constructive solutions.

An ultrasound examination can be rather long, and if possible, attractive decor can help minimize the patient's awareness of discomfort. The room should be large enough to accomodate a standard static B-scanner with arm, an examining stretcher, which will preferably allow the head and feet to be elevated independently, a working desk and chair for the sonographer and a storage area for surgical supplies. One of the laboratory doors should be wide enough to accomodate the critically ill patient in his own hospital bed. If obstetrical and gynecological scans are to be performed, a waiting area with an adjacent rest room must be available. An additional parameter affecting room size will be how many people are directly involved in ultrasound. Usually two ultrasonologists and two sonographers will be on the staff, and with the patient, it is possible that five people plus equipment will be in the room. A safe figure for room size would be no less than 150 square feet, and preferably 15 × 15 feet.

The sonographer can make the every day functioning of the ultrasound laboratory run smoothly by attention to a few pertinent details such as expected case load, type of examination to be performed and additional personnel. The type of examinations to be performed and the balance between inpatient and outpatient work load directly affects patient flow.

For example, if one deals primarily with out-patients, two dressing rooms are advantageous so that one patient can be dressing or undressing while another is being examined. If most patients are inpatients, additional transport facilities may be required as well as a stretcher waiting area which allows continued observation.

The following is a list of examinations currently being performed at this hospital:

Abdomen: Complete, or limited, involving aorta, retroperitoneum, gallbladder, liver, pancreas, kidney, adrenals, spleen, urinary bladder, pelvic masses.

OB/GYN: Complete pregnancy, molar pregnancy, ectopic/intrauterine pregnancy diagnosis, IUD localization, pelvic mass, fetal cephalometry, amniocentesis.

Special Examinations: Thyroid, prostate, cyst puncture, skinny needle biopsy, pleural effusion aspiration, chest wall thickness and port evaluation for radiation therapy, Baker's cysts, superficial lesions, abscess localization, breast scanning.

Cardiology: M-mode, real-time.

While this list will certainly enlarge as the applications for diagnostic ultrasound grow, it supplies the sonographer with a good idea of what type of case load can be expected.

To expedite good patient care, a memorandum should be prepared for distribution to patient floors and all interested clinicians, announcing the availability of ultrasound and containing all necessary information they will need. Include the following main points in this memorandum. List all telephone numbers, location and hours of operation of the ultrasound laboratory. Give a short introduction of the personnel associated with the service. Describe all preparations necessary for patients undergoing ultrasound examination, specifically, the necessity for a full urinary bladder for OB/GYN studies and instructions for fasting for upper abdominal examinations. This is also a good time to explain why ultrasound examination must be performed prior to barium studies. Explain what forms to use when ordering examinations. Include the list of examinations available and an explanation of when and where reports on examinations

can be obtained. At this institution a "wet reading" book is completed at the time of interpretation and the results recorded. This book is available after hours so that official results are available for the referring physician at all times, prior to receiving a fully typed report. Ideally all inpatients should have a written report entered in their charts at the time of examination, but in practice this may prove to be difficult.

It is not possible for an ultrasonographer to see a full day's schedule of patients and still answer the telephone to schedule patients and give reports. A receptionist is especially necessary when a large share of the case load involves outpatients. However, the sonographer should always speak with the referring clinician if any specific difficulties in the case are anticipated. Quite often, the receptionist is required to give verbal reports over the phone and this necessitates a familiarity with contemporary ultrasound jargon.

Because ultrasound continues to be primarily a non-invasive diagnostic procedure, very ill patients, too sick to tolerate other procedures, are often referred for examination, and the possibility of cardiac or respiratory arrest is always present. The sonographer has direct responsibility to see that all the necessary emergency apparatus is available. Routine refresher courses in CPR for all staff will help keep everyone prepared for such possibilities.

An ever-expanding use of ultrasound in the emergency situation necessitates some form of emergency coverage for the ultrasound department. The diagnosis of acute cholelithiasis, ectopic pregnancy, bleeding during pregnancy, pericardial effusion, the post-surgical patient with fever of undetermined origin, abdominal aortic aneurysm, exclusion of hydronephrosis in the patient with a history of iodine intolerance or an elevated BUN and acute pancreatic disease are representative of the steadily growing list of emergency ultrasound examinations.

The care of the emergency patient at night is an important ethical situation. Unlike those who work with other imaging disciplines, the sonographer is intimately involved in obtaining a diagnosis. Consequently he or she has a responsibility to alert the physician when a life-threatening situation is encountered. Examples would include a large, unsuspected abdominal aortic aneurysm, or discovery of a retroperitoneal bleed in a patient with a steadily falling hematocrit. This responsibility also applies in day-to-day work, but becomes more critical in the off-duty time period.

The sonographer is often the first to examine a patient during a stay in the hospital and is in a position to foster a pleasant and positive attitude for the patient. The American Institute of Ultrasound in Medicine as well as several commercial manufacturers produce pamphlets on ultrasound, and these are helpful in alleviating the patient's anxiety about the examination. Once the patient is in the examining room, the question may arise as to whether close family should be present. Expectant mothers often request that their spouses be permitted to watch. Though each individual situation is unique, the sonographer must realize that occasionally unsuspected problems are uncovered and often the explanation of the examination results requires great tact. When the question of twins exists, it is best to coax a response from the mother concerning this possibility before the examination is begun. This will often provide a key to how much information can be safely discussed. Many sonographers give photographs of the fetus to the mother. This is best done only on request, and is becoming more difficult with the growing use of multiformat cameras.

The problem of discussing the patient's condition during the examination can be a stumbling block in patient care. The sonographer and ultrasonologist must develop a second language between them; a form of conversation that gives the patient the least anxiety. The inter-relationship of organ systems as visualized by ultrasound require a certain amount of open discussion during the examination to ensure that all areas are examined thoroughly. Ultrasound has developed a language of its own. The use of this terminology will enable the examiners to avoid mentioning specific disease processes.

If the ultrasonologist is unable to see the patient with a particularly involved medical picture, the sonographer's presence at the afternoon read-out session can be most helpful. Additionally, a common nomenclature for the labelling of scanning planes will make the scans more readable. Newer pieces of equipment have the convenience of built-in patient locators, but they often do not compensate for the unique projections necessary to define a specific organ. Only in the establishment of ports for radiation therapy, and subsequent monitoring of tumor regression are precise calculations of planes required.

When compared with other diagnostic imaging techniques, ultrasound still remains in its infancy. Consequently the need for continuing education in the ultrasound laboratory is vital. All sonographers have a committment to obtain national registries for the areas in which they work. Due to the newness of the modality, the sonographer is often called upon to teach as well as perform ultrasound. Many seminars, workshops and lectures are held throughout the year, as well as two national meetings sponsored by the American Intitute of Ultrasound in Medicine and the American Society of Ultrasound Technical Specialists. Current literature, in the form of books, journals and articles, should be available to people with an interest in ultrasound.

If the facility has an ongoing radiologic technician program, arrangements can be made to allow students to rotate through the ultrasound section for a minimum period of one month. Many times, a small general quiz at the end of each rotation increases attentiveness and encourages the student to pursue further ultrasound studies.

Diagnostic ultrasound, like many medical imaging modalities, is undergoing substantial growth and consequently is a field inundated by many new advances in instrumentation. Sonographers are obligated to stay abreast of current advances in instrumentation, and be able to estimate where each advance may be applicable in their own laboratories. One of the parameters for diagnostic success in a laboratory is the ability to recognize the interchangable nature of ultrasound modalities as the specific need arises. The use of A-mode to differentiate the contents of a renal cyst that is confusing on standard B-scans, M-mode in the obstetrical study to document fetal viability, and the use of real-time to separate an abscess from normal bowel with peristalsis are but a few of the examples of using complementary techniques. Much of this information has been discussed in detail in the preceding chapters on physics and instrumentation. However, an overview of the individual controls, with emphasis on how they affect scanning is helpful at this point. While equipment may vary from manufacturer to manufacturer, all units provide functions which are manipulated by a series of common controls. Each function will be discussed separately.

TGC (Time Gain Compensation) allows the sonographer to produce realistic tissue images and to obtain uniform tissue texture, independent of the natural attenuation of the body. The TGC is controlled through three adjustments: initial, slope and far gain. Individual settings for the TGC, as they apply to specific organs, have been discussed in previous chapters (pp. 11 – 12). However, there are no absolute settings for any particular examination, and the sonographer must appreciate what is unique to the particular equipment employed. A rule of thumb is to adjust the 'knee' of the slope just past the point of interest, then adjust the initial gain to a depth that does not overwrite the near field.

Power, input/output, gain, attenuation. These terms are all synonomous for the control which affects the overall image by controlling the power applied directly to the transducer. This control should be adjusted to a level which realistically demonstrates solid/cystic interfaces. On most equipment, this adjustment is made after the TGC has been established.

A-, B-, M- display selection. All units should have a selection switch for the display of A-, B-, or M-mode. They are usually displayed on different oscilloscopes at different times. Often obtaining a diagnosis is directly dependent on the sonographer's ability to interchange between these modes freely. To date, the A-mode remains the most sensitive.

Survey, stepping, slew. Most units supply some type of control over the movement of the scanning arm. Survey, stepping and slew are the more common terms for this control. Many sonographers, however, find these preset arm speeds too slow and may choose to move the arm through some other independent means. Preset arm movement offers increased accuracy in the scan but hampers the speed with which a scan may be completed.

Character generator. Character generators are electronic keyboards which allow information (patient's name, identification number, date, and scan position) to be entered on the television and become part of the permanent record when the image is photographed. They represent a valuable complement to ultrasound scanning and may be either free standing or built into the control panel of the unit. Most character generators utilize a standard typewriter format.

Calipers markers, digital calipers. All units are equipped with some means of obtaining accurate measurements. This may take the form of a bar graph, centimeter/millimeter dots, or digital calipers. All will adjust automatically to the scale selection. Digital calipers are the most useful since they give a digital display of the actual measurement and may be easily placed anywhere on the image. If digital calipers are not employed, common drawing dividers should be supplied in the laboratory and reading area for the purpose of transferring measurements.

Image format reversal. Image format reversal refers to the use of either a white background with black writing or a black background with white writing. Some interesting work is currently in progress concerning the perceptual advantages of each of these formats. Currently, all work at this institution is being done on a black background with white writing. However, the ultimate choice lies with the individual responsible for interpretation.

Gray-scale/bistable selection. This switch is self explanatory and merely indicates the program selection within which you may operate. The origins of this control are explained in detail in the chapter on Instrumen-

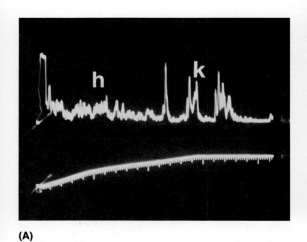
(A)

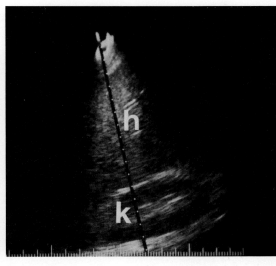
(B)

Fig. 4-1. **(A)** and **(B)** B-scan with corresponding A-mode. H = Liver, K = Kidney.

tation. Currently, bistable mode is used only for obtaining biparietal diameters, establishing radiation therapy ports and defining the internal contents of cysts.

Survey/write/erase. This modality allows the operator to write and erase spontaneously. It is primarily applicable to quick survey scanning over an area of interest, i.e., gallbladder. However, image quality is degraded in this format, and final photography should not be performed in this mode. This mode can also be used to designate a certain area of a standard B-scan for A-mode analysis (Fig. 4-1A and B).

The ideas and principles which apply to setting up a static scanner for operation apply equally well to real-time equipment, with many of the controls overlapping.

Transducers

With the advent of digital processing in static B-scanners, most abdominal examinations are now being performed using a frequency of 3.5 MHz. Frequencies as low as 1.6 MHz are seldom used. Another advance which has improved the overall image quality has been the introduction of transducers with quarter wave length matching layers, discussed previously (pp. 13–15).

Each laboratory must have a good selection of transducers available to handle the wide variations in body habitus. The following transducers should cover all extremes for cardiac testing:

2.25 MHz MIF (medium internal focus)
3.5 MHz MIF
2.25 MHz LIF (long internal focus)

For abdominal investigations, this group of transducers will prove adequate:

2.25 MHz LIF
1.6 MHz LIF
3.5 MHz MIF
2.25 MHz biopsy (slot or doughnut)
5.0 MHz MIF

Calibration of transducers insures that there is no gradual loss of resolution. The transducers should not be jarred or dropped, as this will cause them to depolarize and form side lobes. A simple and quick method used to qualitate transducer performance is to use a one inch plexiglass block as a test object. A block in test position is shown in Figure 4-2A, and the resulting A-mode in Figure 4-2B. The spikes should be adjusted so that there is no blunting of the peaks. This test is done with the TGC turned completely off. The power/output is recorded along with a photograph of the A-mode, and any variations from this

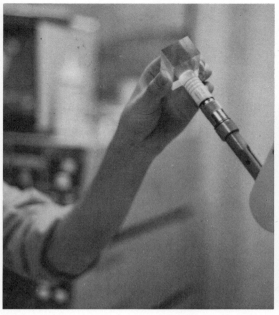

(A)

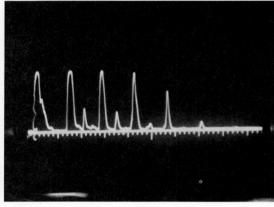

(B)

Fig. 4-2. **(A)** Test block in position. **(B)** Resulting A-mode.

original will give a quick indication of potential problems.

Another, more elaborate testing system, is the use of the standard 100 mm test object, shown in Figure 4-3. Adopted by the American Institute of Ultrasound in Medicine as the official test standard, it offers the users of ultrasound equipment a chance to assess a variety of transducer functions, such as vertical linearity, axial and depth resolution, power

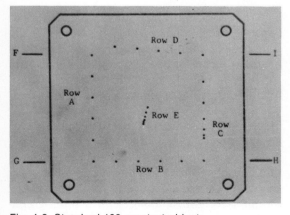

Fig. 4-3. Standard 100 mm test object.

output, beam focus and dead zone. Once the initial test procedures are completed, follow-up tests can be performed in a relatively short period of time.

Photography

With all the recent advances made in the field of ultrasound imaging, the final result submitted for interpretation can be no better than the photographic method used to record it. Various contemporary recording methods will be discussed here, along with some of their advantages and limitations.

Three camera systems handle most of the abdominal and OB/GYN scanning being performed today. These are the Polaroid camera, which provides an immediate viewing capacity; the multiformat camera, using 8 × 10 film and offering a selection of 4,6,9,or 16 images per sheet of film; and the roll film back, which is capable of producing 70,90 and 105 mm images.

Polaroid, in addition to regular black and white film, offers an instant film with a negative and an 8 × 10 film with cassettes which will fit most multiformat cameras and are designed for daylight loading and developing. Instant film is limited by inherent short scale of contrast, and is also rather cost prohibitive. It is important to have an instant camera available though, to provide permanent chart copies, teaching file copies, etc.

The multiformat camera and the roll film back increase the excellence of the final image. There is much greater latitude in film selection, clear base vs. blue base, and a variety of speeds and grains to choose from. Single emulsion mammography film is good to begin with, offering both a long scale of contrast and a reasonable exposure time. We feel that 16 images on an 8 × 10 film is excessive; nine images are suitable for obstetrics, but information on the detailed anatomy of the upper abdomen is lost. We therefore use a six image format.

If either roll or sheet transparancies are employed, dark room and developing facilities will be needed in close proximity to the examining area. This is especially important to reduce the amount of time that a patient must be left alone. Viewboxes should be available in both the examining and reading areas. Some units now offer 32 different gray levels, which can only be realized with a film offering a long scale of contrast. In addition, transparencies are easier to copy than Polaroid film. The choice of a recording medium is mainly one of convenience vs. quality. Regardless of which medium is chosen, two sets of exposure factors must be calculated to provide for white on black, and black on white images.

Standard M-mode is recorded on either a Polaroid (limited sweep) film, or on some type of recording paper. This paper is activated by either light or heat. The light-sensitive paper seems to be easier and more reliable to work with, but either type can be copied, folded and stored with relative ease.

Real-time equipment requires the use of some type of taping device to record final images. One-half or three-quarter inch video tape systems work well, offering up to four hours of taping as well as easy review. However, three-quarter inch tapes offer significantly better reproduction. Cassette recording systems are available which allow for review through the ultrasound monitor. Adaptations can also be made between the video tape equipment and the ultrasound monitor to allow for stopped frame photography. It is a good idea to keep enough blank tapes on hand so that original studies can be kept for a period of time without being re-recorded.

5

Obstetrics

KENNETH J. W. TAYLOR
PAULA JACOBSON

INTRODUCTION

Obstetrics is the oldest and most accepted application for diagnostic ultrasound. It has been used since the pioneering studies of Professor Ian Donald in Glasgow in 1955. Using older bistable machines, multiple gestation, fetal presentation, maturity and placental localization could all be diagnosed. These four aspects of an obstetric ultrasound examination still remain the most important ones; but the more sophisticated instrumentation currently employed permits display of the detailed anatomy of the fetus so that the prenatal diagnosis of fetal abnormality is possible. With increasing experience, complications of pregnancy are more easily recognized.

NORMAL FETAL DEVELOPMENT

Gestational age is dated from the commence-ment of the last menstrual period (LMP). Since ovulation does not usually occur until the 14th day of the menstrual cycle, the true period of gestation is two weeks less than that given by obstetric tables. For uniformity with other obstetric data, maturity determined from nomograms of ultrasonic parameters refers to the gestational age from last menstrual period.

As early as four weeks after the last menstrual period, a gestational sac is seen in utero. At this time, no fetal parts may be seen. The sac can be measured as a parameter of fetal maturity but is less accurate than the later crown-to-rump measurements. At six weeks, fetal parts are visualized, and at eight weeks the fetal heart can be detected by M-mode or A-mode examination. Crown-to-rump measurements can be made at this point and are accurate to within three days. The fetal head can frequently be seen by eight or nine weeks gestation, but nomograms for biparietal diameter are not available before 12 weeks. In early gestation, the placenta may surround the entire uterine volume and is referred to as a *"wrap around"* placenta.

SCANNING TECHNIQUE

The pregnant patient must present for examination with a full urinary bladder. This is essential in the first trimester to displace air-containing gut lying anterior to the uterus. In later pregnancy, the bladder does not have to be exceptionally full, but some distention of the bladder lifts the fetal head out of the pelvis and permits visualization of the cervix. With the cervix visualized, the precise relationship between the lower edge of the placenta and the cervix can be established. Over-distention of the bladder may produce the appearance of a placenta previa; this point will be discussed later.

The obstetric patient lies supine on the examining table. Occasionally, she may complain of faintness during the examination and this is due to the weight of the uterus on the inferior vena cava which obstructs venous return. If this happens, the examination must be suspended and the patient told to turn over to her left or right side; there will be almost immediate recovery.

Mineral oil is liberally applied over the anterior abdominal wall to provide a coupling medium. The choice of transducer frequency depends on the stage of gestation, the size of the patient and the sensitivity of the equipment. In early gestation, 3.5 MHz or even 5 MHz can be used, while in late pregnancy and in large patients, a frequency of 2.25 MHz must be employed. The midline sagittal plane is scanned with a long sector scan from the pelvis to display the cervix, continuing into a linear scan up to the fundus of the uterus. Virtually no compound scanning should be used because significant fetal movement obscures details when multiple registrations are made. Adjustment of TGC and overall gain are necessary to compensate for tissue attenuation. The TGC is correctly set when both the anterior and posterior uterine structures are equally written. The presence of amniotic fluid, which has virtually zero attenuation, may render this difficult. When the beam passes through a large pocket of amniotic fluid, there may be some overwriting of the distal structures if the TGC is set to compensate for soft tissue attenuation. The amniotic cavity is immediately apparent on both the A-scan and the B-scan because of the absence of echoes. The scanning arm is then moved continually to the left and then to the right while multiple scans are made in the paramedian plane. This is an overall screening procedure which permits determination of the number of fetuses and their overall lie. It also permits immediate localization of the bulk of the placenta. The sonographer should then turn the scanning arm through a right angle to scan transversely in the parasagittal plane. Serial sections should be made with the arm in continuous motion from the pelvis to the fundus of the uterus. The sonographer must have the ability to integrate serial sections into a three dimensional image.

At the end of this screening procedure, the sonographer should be aware of the position of the fetus, the number of fetuses, and the position of the bulk of the placenta. Careful and thorough sections are now taken for permanent recording purposes. The initial screening can be performed using a real-time system. Because of the large acoustic window available, the linear arrays are economic and effective ways of carrying out this initial screening. However, for the purposes of record-taking, we still prefer manual sections using a static B-scanner, because at present this provides higher resolution than that available on any real-time system.

PRESENTATION OF FETUS

The scanning arm is replaced in the midline sagittal plane and a slow static section taken. After 34 weeks gestation approximately 90 percent of fetuses are in the vertex presentation (Fig. 5-1). Before this date, the fetus may be in any presentation and indeed, in the second trimester (12-24 weeks), the fetus is extremely active and may reverse its position

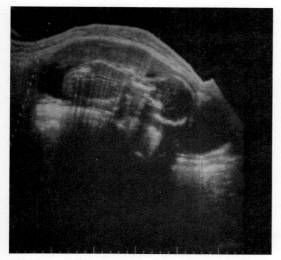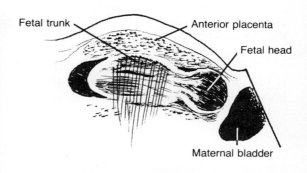

Fig. 5-1. Longitudinal scan. The fetal head is inferior and in close proximity to the maternal bladder. An anterior placenta is seen.

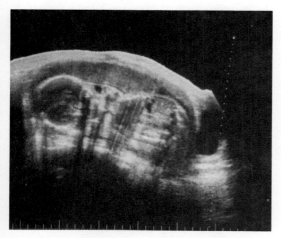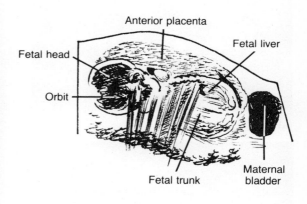

Fig. 5-2. Longitudinal scan of fetus in breech presentation. The fetal head is seen in the fundus of the uterus. An anterior placenta is seen.

many times during the ultrasound examination. It is under these conditions, in particular, that a real-time machine, such as a linear array, is invaluable to exclude the presence of twins, rather than taking multiple images of one rapidly moving fetus.

In patients who have had many children (multiparae), the anterior abdominal wall may be flaccid and lack adequate musculature, so that the fetal head may lie high even to term. In the woman who has had fewer children, the fetal head is normally engaged in the pelvis by 34-36 weeks. This may produce difficulty in measuring biparietal diameter if the bladder is not filled to displace the fetal head from the deep pelvis.

The second most common lie is breech presentation, and this accounts for approximately 10 percent of presentations at term (Fig. 5-2). Breech presentation is usually detected by clinical palpation except in the obese patient and is confirmed by ultrasound examination. An important aspect of the ultrasound examination is the further search for abnormality that may be the cause for breech presentation. These include disproportion, fetal abnormality and a mass in the lower portion of the uterus, such as placenta previa, fibroid or a twin fetus.

Disproportion occurs when the fetal head is too large for the maternal pelvis, thereby preventing engagement of the head into the pelvis and spontaneous vaginal delivery. Disproportion is relative, that is, it depends on the size of the maternal pelvis compared with that of the fetal head, so that there are no absolute measurements which imply that the fetus is too large for spontaneous vaginal delivery. The size of the fetal head and the pelvic capacity can be approximately estimated and these figures are supplemented by clinical examination. The fetal head may be pathologically

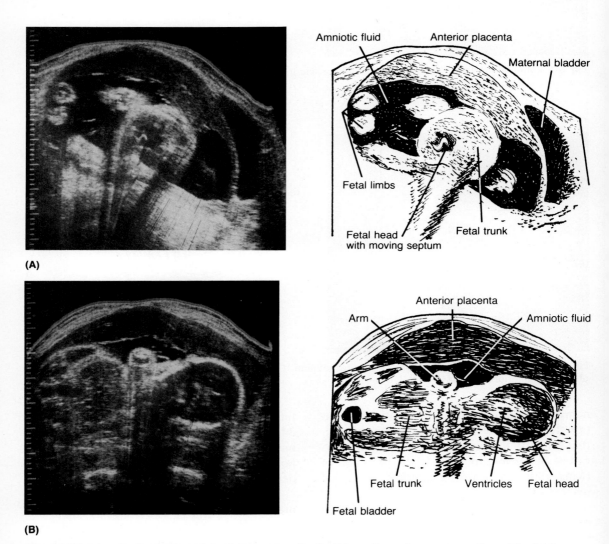

(A)

(B)

Fig. 5-3 **(A)** A longitudinal scan of fetus in transverse lie. On this section a transverse section of the fetal thorax is seen, including the fetal heart. An anterior placenta is seen. **(B)** Transverse section showing fetus in transverse lie. The fetal head and trunk are seen in the transverse plane.

large, for example in the case of pronounced postmaturity or hydrocephaly. Hydocephaly (p. 80) is reliably diagnosed by ultrasound. Other fetal abnormalities such as anencephaly or meningomyelocele may also produce sufficient distortion of the external contour of the fetus and cause breech presentation.

The presence of a mass in the lower segment of the uterus must be excluded by ultrasound examination. Placenta previa is usually apparent (see below); a supracervical fibroid or other pelvic tumor must be excluded. Finally, a twin must be excluded since the most common position for twins is one in the vertex and one in breech presentation.

Other presentations include pure transverse (Fig. 5-3A and B) and various oblique presentations. All such presentations are abnormal and are incompatable with normal spontaneous delivery if they persist to term.

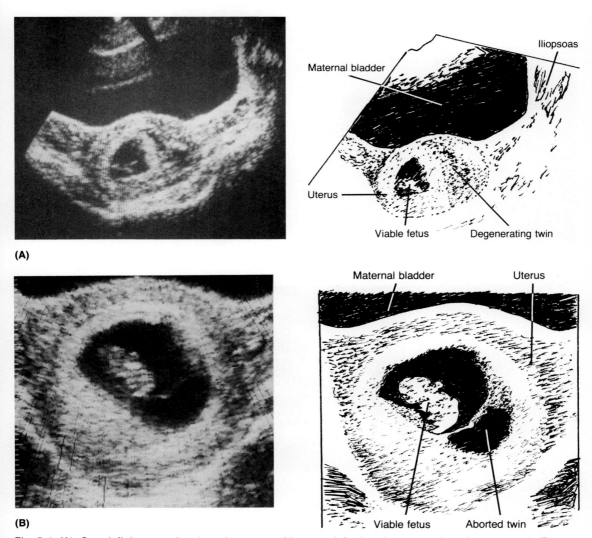

Fig. 5-4. **(A).** One definite gestational sac is seen on this scan. A further degenerated sac is also noted. **(B)** Magnified image of uterus containing one viable fetus and missed abortion twin. The second fetal sac is in the process of being reabsorbed.

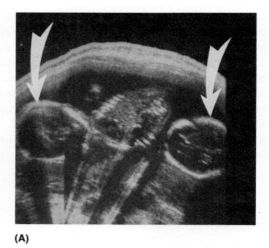

(A)

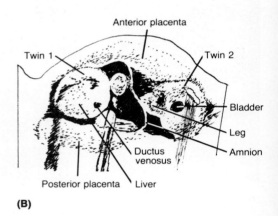

(B)

(B)

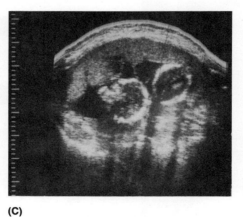

(C)

Fig. 5-5 **(A)** Longitudinal section showing twins, one in vertex presentation and the other in breech presentation. The fetal heads (arrowed) are seen at opposite ends of the uterus. **(B)** Transverse section through twins. Note that the midabdomen is cut on one twin and the pelvis cut on the other. The twins are separated by the amnion. Each twin has its own placenta and this indicates that these are dissimilar (dizygotic) twins. **(C)** Transverse section at a level just below the symphysis pubis showing twin gestation; both twins are in vertex presentation. Sections through both fetal heads are seen.

As with breech presentations, the cause of malpresentation should be sought. It must be stressed again that in early pregnancy any of these presentations may occur and the fetus moves rapidly from one presentation to another, so that at up to 30 weeks, presentation has no meaning as far as the definitive position is concerned.

Multiple Gestation

Twin gestation occurs in 1/80 live pregnancies and triplets 1/6400. However, the true incidence may be greater than this since the presence of multiple gestational sacs with subsequent disappearance at a later date have been noted (Fig. 5-4A and B). The sonographer

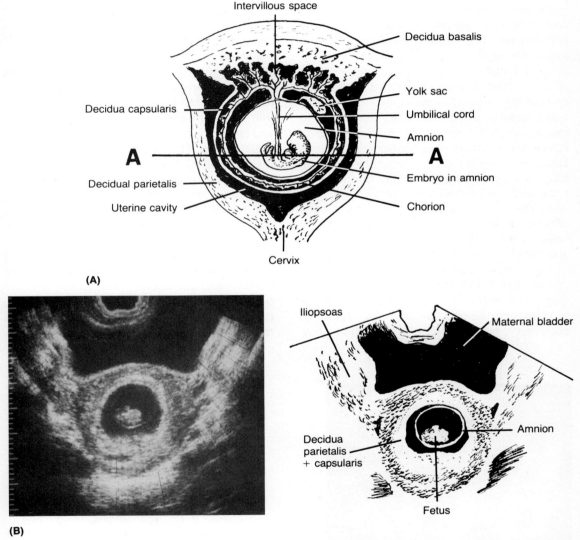

Fig. 5-6 **(A)** Schema to show early development of decidua and membranes in the second month of pregnancy. The decidua basalis is the site of the future placenta and the embryonic villi extend into this area to obtain nutrition. The embryo is seen suspended by the umbilical cord in the amniotic cavity. The uterine cavity is still seen between the decidua parietalis and decidua capsularis, and menstrual loss may continue from this until the deciduae fuse at approximately 12 weeks and obliterate the uterine cavity. **(B)** Transverse ultrasound section taken through the plane indicated by line A——A. The embryo is seen within its amniotic cavity and the decidual layers are seen forming the so-called gestational ring.

should be familiar with the drug Clomid, which is a gonadotropin used to treat infertility. The effect of this drug is somewhat unpredictable and multiple gestations with it are extremely common. In one such patient, we observed three gestational sacs at six weeks, which reduced to one within one month — much to the parents' relief! Thus, there is probably a higher incidence of twin and triplet gestations than previously considered, with reabsorption of one fetus in a number of these pregnancies. The major difficulty for the sonographer in diagnosing multiple gestations is actually counting fetal heads in the presence of very active fetuses. Prior to the development of high resolution real-time systems, this was a major problem, solved by attempting to image both fetal heads in the same plane. With active fetuses this was rather challenging. However, with the use of linear arrays, each fetus is easily imaged, and the sonographer can rapidly move the transducer over the uterus to ensure that an accurate count has been effected. This is especially important when a large number of fetuses is present such as quintuplets and sextuplets.

The most common position for twins is one in breech and one in vertex presentation (Fig. 5-5A and B). However, one twin may be in transverse lie and the other in vertex, or both may be in vertex presentation (Fig. 5-5C). With triplets almost any position of the fetuses may occur.

Placental Localization

Placental localization is important to exclude placenta previa. Clinical suspicion of placenta previa occurs either because of bleeding in early pregnancy, or because of persistent malpresentation close to term. To appreciate the different appearances during pregnancy, it is necessary to review the development of the placenta.

The ovum is fertilized in the Fallopian tubes and commences cell division. Three or four days after fertilization, it arrives in the uterine lumen, the walls of which are vascular and spongy in the secretory phase of the menstrual cycle. The embryo now burrows into the wall and with this implantation, the site of the future placenta is determined. The endometrium of the uterus is known as the decidua and is subdivided as shown in Figure 5-6A and B. The decidua on the superficial surface of the embryo is called the *decidua capsularis,* that on the distal wall of the uterus is called the *decidua parietalis,* and that between the embryo and the uterine wall is the *decidua basalis.* With subsequent growth of the fetus, the decidua capsularis and parietalis fuse, and the uterine cavity is thereby obliterated. Be-

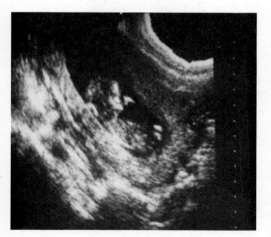
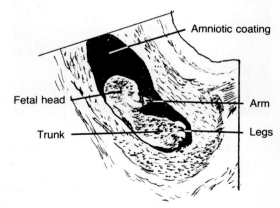

Fig. 5-7. Longitudinal section through an early gestational sac showing a fetus in crown-to-rump extent. Notice that the fetal head, trunk and limbs can easily be seen at this stage, and fetal heart motion can be verified.

cause of the persistence of a uterine cavity for approximately the first 12 weeks of pregnancy, menstrual bleeding can occur from this lumen, and this is a frequent source of confusion as to the maturity of the fetus. The decidua basalis is the site of the future placenta.

In early gestation the placenta may appear to be wrap-around in type (Fig. 5-7), that is, without specific localization on the uterine wall. Because of variations during the course of pregnancy, it is pointless to comment on placental position until the third trimester, unless the placenta is almost entirely central previa (Fig. 5-8). Due to the massive growth of the uterine wall, the area of the uterine wall which is occupied by the placenta becomes progressively smaller. The placenta may be predominantly anterior (Fig. 5-9), posterior (Fig. 5-10), fundal (Fig. 5-11) or spread over two or more walls. However, the most important aspect of the sonographer's duty is to display the relation of the placenta to the internal uterine os.

An important phenomenon known as *migration* of the *placenta* should now be considered. Migration of the placenta produces considerable confusion and currently some

controversy. First, it is quite obvious that the placenta is connected to the uterine wall for the entire pregnancy, and that there will be no shift of the placenta relative to the uterine wall which is deep to it at any time during gesta-

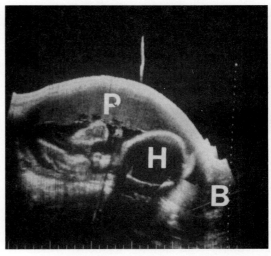

Fig. 5-9. Longitudinal midline scan showing anterior placenta. The placenta (P) is seen entirely on the anterior wall extending from the fundus to the region of the symphysis pubis. The fetal head (H) is seen below this and in proximity to the maternal bladder (B).

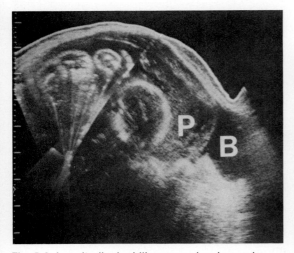

Fig. 5-8. Longitudinal midline scan showing major degree of placenta previa. The placenta (P) is in immediate proximity to the maternal bladder (B) and the edge of the placenta covers the cervix. There are degenerative changes in the placenta indicating approaching maturity.

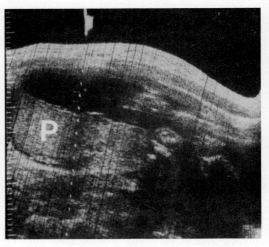

Fig. 5-10. Longitudinal scan showing posterior placenta. The placenta (P) is seen on the posterior wall of the uterus extending down from the fundus.

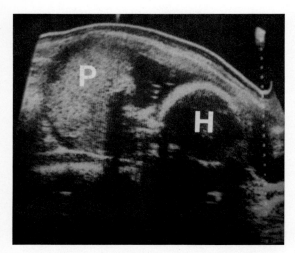

Fig. 5-11. Longitudinal midline scan showing fundal placenta. A bulky placenta (P) is seen occupying the fundus of the uterus with the fetal head (H) situated inferiorly, indicating vertex presentation.

tion. However, the uterine wall is dynamic, particularly the lower segment which is formed by the muscle which comprises the cervix in the nonpregnant state. Thus, if the placenta is low early in pregnancy, but the cervix is subsequently spread into a thin uterine wall forming most of the lower part of the uterus, the net effect will be a movement of the placenta upwards, away from the cervix. Because of this relative migration of the placenta, if it appears to be low at 26 weeks (Fig. 5-12A), the scans should be repeated later in pregnancy when the placenta may well have cleared the lower segment of the uterus (Fig. 5-12B).

Some researchers have demonstrated the occurence of migration by review of old arteriography studies; others have shown that overdistention of the urinary bladder may cause an anterior placenta to appear previa. If the urinary bladder displaces the lower uterine wall into apposition with the placenta, it appears that the placenta has a lower origin than is actually the case (Fig. 5-13A). When the bladder is empty, the uterine wall, which is in fact free of placental origins, descends and its freedom from the placenta is more apparent (Fig. 5-13B). Extreme views have been voiced which suggest that all placental migration is

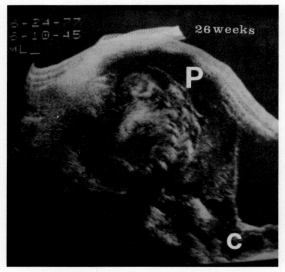

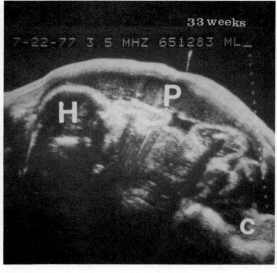

(A)   (B)

Fig. 5-12. Apparent migration of the placenta. (A) At 26 weeks the placenta (P) is seen to be situated low on the anterior wall of the uterus, with the lower edge close to the cervix (C). (B) A repeat scan at 33 weeks shows the placenta concentrated entirely on the anterior wall of the uterus, with a considerable interval between the lower margin of the placenta (P) and the cervix (C). Note that the fetal head (H) is in the fundus of the uterus, indicating a breech presentation.

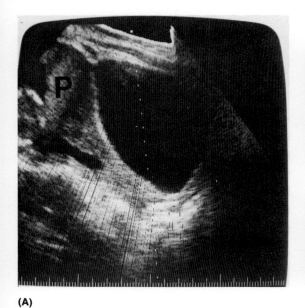

(A)

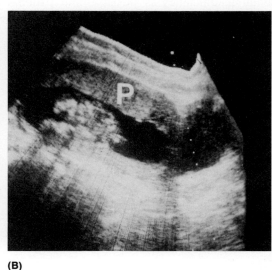

(B)

Fig. 5-13 **(A).** Spurious placenta previa due to full bladder. **(B)** Apparent placenta previa. The placenta (P) appears low lying with the bladder full. But with an empty bladder, the true lower edge of the placenta is seen to be well clear of the cervix.

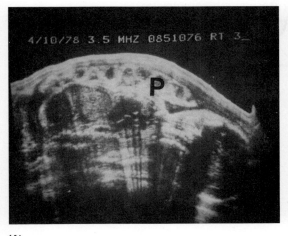

(A)

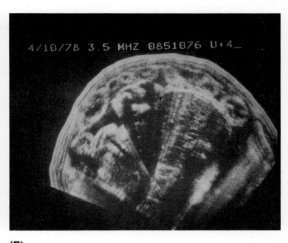

(B)

Fig. 5-14. **(A)** Longitudinal and **(B)** transverse scans to show changes of placental maturity.

artifactual due to this displacement of the lower uterine wall by a filled urinary bladder. This is clearly fallacious since there is uptake of the cervix to form the lower segment, and there is excellent arteriographic evidence to support the concept of placental migration. Again, the practical point must be stressed that the definitive position of the placenta should be established in patients with questionable placenta previa at 36 weeks gestation or later, when placental maturity begins in the normal pregnancy. More homogeneous areas are seen with high level echoes around the cotyledons (Fig. 5-14A and B). When the placenta shows premature maturity changes, placental insufficiency is possible and patients are frequently hypertensive. Placental insufficiency may result in intrauterine growth retardation (see pp. 79–80).

Determination of Fetal Maturity

The determination of fetal maturity is one of the most important aspects of obstetrical examination. With the large numbers of the population on contraceptive pills, the date of the last menstrual period is frequently erroneous. Patients may also have scant menses during the first one to three months of pregnancy, for reasons discussed above. On the other hand, patients may bleed because of threatened abortion or may abort and become pregnant again. For all these reasons, gestational age based on the date of the last menstrual period may be incorrect. The most accurate technique for the estimation of gestational age is based on crown-to-rump measurement as described by Robinson. With the increasing availability of high resolution real-time systems, crown-to-rump measurement is more easily determined. Hitherto, attempting to define the precise crown-to-rump axis of a highly mobile fetus was time consuming and not always practical. The crown-to-rump measurement (Fig. 5-7) allows an estimation of maturity accurate to within three days. Crown-to-rump measurements for the first 14 weeks of gestation are shown in Table 5-1. From 12 weeks, the biparietal measurement is feasible, although again, because of

TABLE 5-1. CROWN-RUMP MEASUREMENT AS A DETERMINANT OF FETAL AGE. THIS DETERMINATION IS A USEFUL AND SENSITIVE INDICATOR OF GESTATIONAL AGE. IN VERY EARLY PREGNANCY SOME PATIENCE IS REQUIRED TO OBTAIN THE PROPER PLANE FOR MEASUREMENT.

Menstrual Maturity (weeks + days)	CRL (mm) Mean	CRL (mm) 2 S.D.	Menstrual Maturity (weeks + days)	CRL (mm) Mean	CRL (mm) 2 S.D.
6 + 2	7.0	3.3	10 + 0	33.0	7.2
6 + 3	6.5	1.4	10 + 1	33.8	7.6
6 + 4	7.0·	4.6	10 + 2	35.2	7.3
6 + 5	6.5	4.2	10 + 3	36.0	7.9
6 + 6	10.0	2.6	10 + 4	37.3	9.7
7 + 0	9.3	2.3	10 + 5	43.4	7.7
7 + 1	10.3	8.0	10 + 6	40.1	7.1
7 + 2	11.8	5.7	11 + 0	46.7	6.1
7 + 3	12.8	4.8	11 + 1	43.6	7.2
7 + 4	13.4	6.7	11 + 2	47.5	6.2
7 + 5	15.4	3.6	11 + 3	48.8	5.9
7 + 6	15.4	4.4	11 + 4	49.0	9.5
8 + 0	17.0	4.9	11 + 5	54.0	9.8
8 + 1	19.5	5.7	11 + 6	56.2	9.5
8 + 2	19.4	6.2	12 + 0	58.3	9.4
8 + 3	20.4	5.0	12 + 1	56.8	7.2
8 + 4	21.3	3.8	12 + 2	59.4	6.6
8 + 5	20.9	2.4	12 + 3	62.6	8.6
8 + 6	23.2	3.6	12 + 4	63.5	9.5
9 + 0	25.8	6.0	12 + 5	67.7	6.4
9 + 1	25.4	4.6	12 + 6	66.5	8.2
9 + 2	26.7	4.4	13 + 0	72.5	4.2
9 + 3	27.0	2.8	13 + 1	69.7	8.5
9 + 4	32.5	4.2	13 + 2	73.0	15.1
9 + 5	30.0	10.0	13 + 3	77.0	8.5
9 + 6	31.3	5.5	13 + 4	—	—
			13 + 5	—	—
			13 + 6	76.0	5.7
			14 + 0	79.6	7.8

(From Robinson, H.P., and Fleming J. E. E.: A critical evaluation of sonar "crown-rump length" measurements. Brit. J. Obstet. Gynaec. 82:702-710, 1975.)

TABLE 5-2. YALE NOMOGRAM FOR BPD USING LEADING EDGE TO LEADING EDGE B-MODE DOTS (GRATICULE) AND BISTABLE GRID

cm	Weeks Gestation Graticule	cm	Weeks Gestation Graticule Grid	cm	Weeks Gestation Graticule
1.9	11.6	4.5	19.9	6.9	28.1
2.0	11.6	4.6	20.4	7.0	28.6
2.1	12.1	4.7	20.4	7.1	29.1
2.2	12.6	4.8	20.9	7.3	29.6
2.3	12.6	4.9	21.3	7.4	30.1
2.4	13.1	5.0	21.3	7.5	30.6
2.5	13.6	5.1	21.8	7.6	31.0
2.6	13.6	5.2	22.3	7.7	31.5
2.7	14.1	5.3	22.3	7.8	32.0
2.8	14.6	5.4	22.8	7.9	32.5
2.9	14.6	5.5	23.3	8.0	33.0
3.0	15.0	5.6	23.3	8.2	33.5
3.1	15.5	5.7	23.8	8.3	34.0
3.2	15.5	5.8	24.3	8.4	34.4
3.3	16.0	5.9	24.3	8.5	34.9
3.4	16.5	6.0	24.7	8.6	35.4
3.5	16.5	6.1	25.2	8.8	35.9
3.6	17.0	6.2	25.2	8.9	36.4
3.7	17.5	6.3	25.7	9.0	36.9
3.8	18.0	6.4	26.2	9.1	37.3
4.0	18.4	6.5	26.2	9.2	37.8
4.2	18.9	6.6	26.7	9.3	*38.3
4.3	19.4	6.7	27.2	9.4	*38.8
4.4	19.4	6.8	27.6	9.6	*39.3
				9.7	*40.0

*indicates a fetus of 36 weeks or greater in a non-diabetic

(Courtesy of John C. Hobbins, M.D., Department of Obstetrics and Gynecology, Yale-New Haven Hospital)

the activity of the fetus, this is a difficult measurement to obtain until approximately 25 weeks. Around this time, an accurate estimation can be obtained since the biparietal diameter is growing rapidly, and the fetus is less active. Because the fetal head grows rapidly up to 30 weeks (up to 4 mm per week), small errors in measurement lead to only a small inaccuracy in gestational age. Towards term, the fetal head grows only 1-2 mm per week (Table 5-2), so that small errors in measurements lead to unacceptable errors in gestational age. Because of this difficulty a precise gestational age after 34 weeks can not be given. The technique for determination of biparietal diameter is detailed in Figure 5-15 A to M.

DETERMINATION OF BIPARIETAL DIAMETER*

Rosie Silverman and K. J. W. Taylor

To determine the biparietal diameter, the gravid uterus is first surveyed to determine the lie of the fetus and the presentation. The plane of the scanning arm is varied until the scan is along the longitudinal axis of the fetal body and head. Next the plane of the skull and cervical spine is identified, since this compensates for any flexion or extension of the cervical spine. When scanning sagittally through the skull, a strong echo is seen which is part of the midline complex. The transducer is placed over this midline echo so that the ultrasound beam is perpendicular to it. The angle between the ultrasound beam and the perpendicular plane is the angle of asynclitism (Fig. 5-15A).

The scanning arm is then rotated through 90 degrees. In the most common vertex pre-

*This section—and Figure 5-15—originally appeared in slightly different form in Taylor, KJW: Atlas of Gray Scale Ultrasonography, p. 322. New York, Churchill Livingstone, 1978.

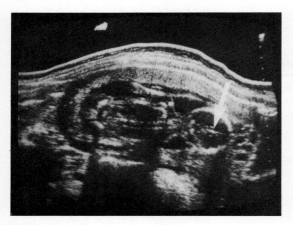

(A)

Fig. 5-15. **(A)** A longitudinal ultrasonogram of a single fetus in vertex presentation shows the position of the midline echo; an arrow represents the ultrasound beam perpendicular to it. The angle between the ultrasound beam and the perpendicular plane is the angle of asynclitism.

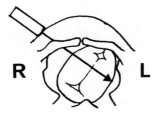

(B)

Fig. 5-15. **(B)** Schema of a fetus in LOA vertex presentation shows plane of scan to identify the longitudinal axis of the head and the position of the ultrasound beam through the biparietal diameter when this is perpendicular to the midline in the correct plane.

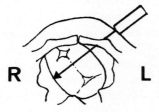

(C)

Fig. 5-15. **(C)** Schema of a fetus in ROA vertex presentation showing plane of scan to identify the longitudinal axis of the head and the position of the ultrasound beam through the biparietal diameter when this is perpendicular to the midline in the correct plane.

sentation, in which the initial scans are carried out in the longitudinal plane, the scanning arm will now be moved into the transverse plane at right angles to the lie of the fetus. The arm is then angled to the same extent as that determined by the angle of asynclitism. A transverse scan is carried out. The skull outline should be oval in shape. The scan is carried out so that the transducer is perpendicular to the long axis of the skull in this plane. The long axis of the skull is determined by compound scans of the skull. The position of the long axis of the skull is shown schematically in Figures 5-15 B and C for LOA and ROA vertex presentations, respectively. In scans in this plane, the anterior horns of both lateral ventricles are seen and the third ventricle is observed in the plane of the biparietal diameter (Fig. 5-15D). The midline echo, which is predominantly from the falx cerebri, should be in the middle of the skull, that is, equidistant from both skull tables (Fig. 5-15E).

If the midline echo is well marked but the third ventricle cannot be seen, the scanning plane is too high on the fetal head and the section is through the crown. If this measurement is taken, it will be smaller than the biparietal diameter.

If the midline echo is of very low amplitude, the lateral ventricles appear very small

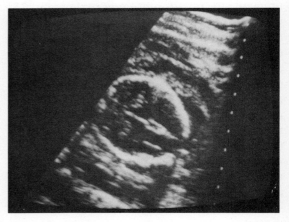

(D)

Fig. 5-15. **(D)** Cross section of fetal head in the biparietal diameter showing the anterior horns of both lateral ventricles and the third ventricle.

or are not seen, and a curved structure is seen on the posterior aspect of the skull, then the scanning plane is too low on the skull. A scan in this plane results in a section through the base of the skull and again is incorrect for the biparietal diameter determination.

If the shape of the skull is not oval (Fig. 5-15F) but appears round or foreshortened, the skull is being scanned obliquely. When such a round contour is seen, the scanning is not truly perpendicular to the longitudinal axis of the fetus. The correct lie of the fetus must be identified and the scanning arm again adjusted to be at right angles to that plane.

If the midline is identified but is not in the middle of the skull, that is, between the two skull tables, the angle of the scanning arm is incorrect. If it is closer to the inferior skull ta-

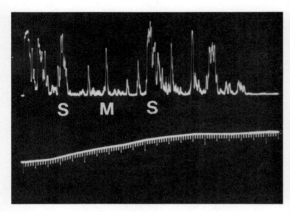

(E)

Fig. 5-15. **(E)** A-mode through biparietal diameter in the plane shown in Figure 5–15B showing the position of the midline (M), which is equidistant from the near and far walls of the skull (S).

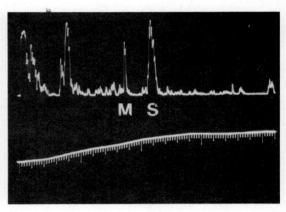

(G)

Fig. 5-15. **(G)** When the ultrasound beam is passed across the fetal head, the midline echo (M) is close to the inferior skull wall (S) and the angle of the scanning arm should be increased.

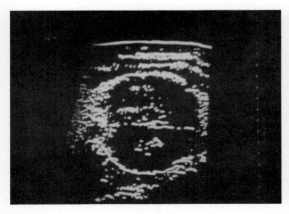

(F)

Fig. 5-15. **(F)** Cross section of fetal skull showing midline, but the scanning plane is not perpendicular to the longitudinal axis of the fetus. Note that this results in a rounded contour for the fetal head.

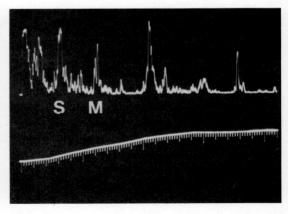

(H)

Fig. 5-15. **(H)** When the ultrasound beam is passed across the fetal head, the midline echo (M) is closer to the nearer skull table (S) and the angle of the scanning arm should be decreased.

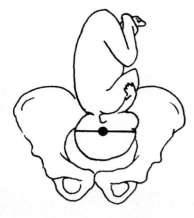

(I)

Fig. 5-15. **(I)** Vertex presentation with flexed head showing plane of biparietal diameter and position of transducer to obtain correct measurements.

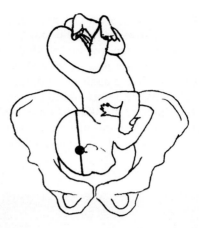

(K)

Fig. 5-15. **(K)** Breech presentation with flexed head showing position of ultrasound beam to obtain correct biparietal diameter.

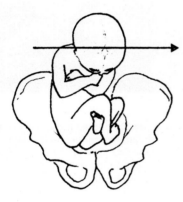

(J)

Fig. 5-15. **(J)** Vertex presentation with fully extended head showing position of biparietal diameter plane and position of ultrasound beam for correct measurement.

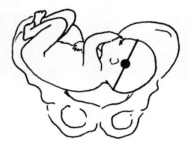

(L)

Fig. 5-15. **(L)** Transverse lie showing position of biparietal diameter and position of ultrasound beam to obtain correct measurement.

ble (Fig. 5-15G), the angle of the scanning arm should be increased. If it is closer to the nearer skull table (Fig. 5-15H), the angle of the scanning arm should be decreased.

The various positions of the fetus are shown in Figures 5-15I – L. They show the fetal head in those positions, and the correct biparietal diameter is shown on each projection. It should be noted that the biparietal diameter passes through the longitudinal axis of the head, which therefore should be oval. The correct biparietal diameter in the bistable

mode is shown in Figure 5-15M. The nomogram for the biparietal diameter in use at Yale is given in Table 5-2. The nomogram was constructed from measurements of the biparietal diameter derived from the bistable oscilloscope screen. The bistable scan has some advantages in that the skull echoes appear thinnest and the measurement made is from the middle of each skull table or from the outer side of the skull table to the inner side of the opposite table. The thicker echoes appearing on the gray scale scan are not easily interpreted in terms of the bistable nomogram. Small differences in the nomograms constructed from different centers, notably those of Camp-

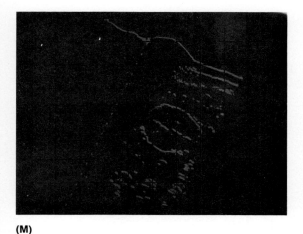

(M)

Fig. 5-15. **(M)** Transverse ultrasonogram of fetal head in bistable mode. Notice that the skull tables appear much thinner and it is easier to obtain an accurate measurement between the cranial walls.

bell in England, can be attributed to the small differences in the velocity of sound which are assumed by Campbell compared with that assumed in the construction of this nomogram. For the calibration of machines used in North America, the nomogram given here is appropriate.

It is technically easiest to estimate the biparietal diameter between 20 and 30 weeks of gestation since the head is easily identified and is relatively round at this period of gestation. After 30 weeks the biparietal eminences become more marked so that the precise biparietal diameter must be recognized; otherwise, there will be a marked inaccuracy in the maturity estimation. Furthermore, the rate at which the biparietal diameter changes after 34 weeks decreases to just over a millimeter per week so that small inaccuracies in the measuring process will lead to large discrepancies in the maturity estimation.

The biparietal diameter should be determined on every fetus before cesarean section to prevent the delivery of a premature infant. For this purpose, a biparietal diameter of 9.3 cm is considered adequate. Fetuses with a biparietal diameter of 9.3 cm seldom present problems with the respiratory distress syndrome, whereas those of lesser maturity may develop significant respiratory problems due to pulmonary immaturity.

NORMAL ANATOMY

Using high quality gray-scale equipment, fetal parts are seen at an early gestational age. The fetal heart chambers are easily delineated (Fig. 5-16A), and fetal heart movement can be monitored either by A-mode, M-mode or on a slow B-scan (Fig. 5-16B). The fetal spine and stomach (Fig. 5-17 A and B), bladder (Fig. 5-18) and kidneys (Fig. 5-19) can also be visualized. Kidney size can be qualitatively assessed on a transverse scan through the fetal abdomen. The kidneys should occupy no more than one-third of the total abdominal area. With real-time equipment, fetal limbs (Fig. 5-20 A and B) can be seen exhibiting movements of increasing complexity with increasing gestational age. The aorta and its bifurcation into the common iliac arteries can be visualized. The coils of the umbilical cord can be seen on many sections, and the entry of the umbilical cord into the fetus is seen on transverse sections. The continuation of the umbilical vein is called the ductus venosus (Fig. 5-17A). For the duration of pregnancy, the ductus venosus shunts blood from the umbilical vein directly into the inferior vena cava, bypassing the liver. The ductus venosus can be seen on transverse sections of the fetal trunk; it forms an important landmark for identifying the midabdominal circumference. Details of the fetal brain and facial skeleton can be displayed (Fig. 5-21). The male genitalia can be seen on an appropriate sector (Fig. 5-22A). The female fetus is recognized by penile absence (Fig. 5-22B). Some authors claim a very high accuracy for correctly determining the sex of the fetus. However, hypertrophy of the clitoris may mimic the penis, and most ultrasonologists do not consider the technique to be sufficiently sensitive to reduce the need for a genetic tap (amniocentesis) when it is important to establish the fetal sex. Fetal sex is important in sex-linked diseases such as hemophilia and sickle cell anemia.

ABNORMALITIES IN PREGNANCY

This text is not intended to cover pathology comprehensively but concentrates on the technique for obtaining scans and details the anatomy with which the sonographer should be familiar. It is, however, important to recog-

nize some common abnormalities so that appropriate scans can be obtained.

Abnormalities in the First Trimester

Uterus Too Large For Dates is commonly caused by incorrect date of LMP,

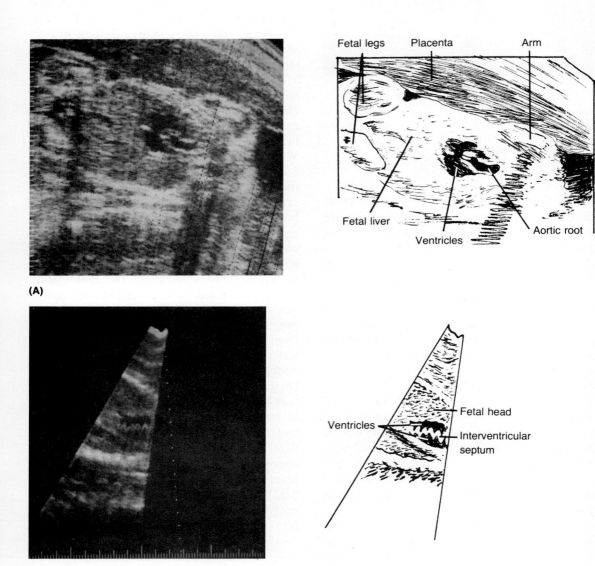

(A)

(B)

Fig. 5-16. **(A).** Longitudinal section through the fetus with a magnified view of the fetal trunk. The aortic root and ventricles are clearly seen. The limbs and fetal trunk are apparent. An anterior placenta is seen. **(B)** Slow B-mode of the heart. The ventricular septum is well seen and the undulations in it are due to ventricular contractions. This verifies fetal viability.

multiple gestation, hydatidiform mole, and co-existing tumor such as a fibroid. The most common cause is an incorrect date of the last menstrual period. Since considerable numbers of the population are on contraceptive pills, the date of the last menstrual period is frequently in error. In these patients accurate dating by crown-to-rump measurements may demonstrate a maturity four weeks different than that based on LMP.

Multiple gestational sacs are easily recognized in the first trimester. A hydatidiform mole can be regarded as a relatively benign tumor arising from the placenta. There is unrestrained growth of the placenta which expands to fill the entire uterine cavity and dis-

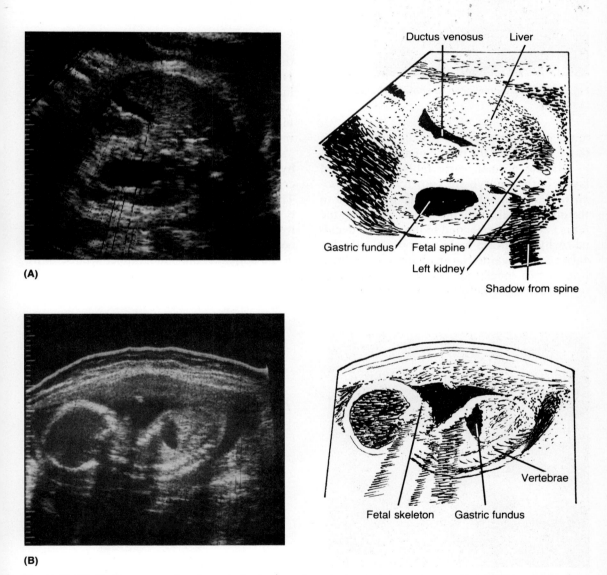

(A)

(B)

Fig. 5-17. **(A).** Transverse section through the fetal trunk at the level of the umbilicus. The ductus venosus is seen passing through the liver substance. At this level, the gastric fundus is seen distended with swallowed amniotic fluid. Fetal spine is seen posteriorly shadowing across the right kidney. **(B)** Fetus in transverse lie. Details of the fetal skull, trunk and abdomen can be visualized. The gastric fundus is well seen as a fluid-filled area. Posteriorly the individual vertebrae can be seen.

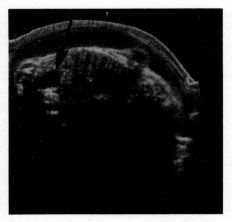

Fig. 5-18. Longitudinal scan to show fetal bladder (arrowed).

tends it to a size that is usually greater than that expected for the period of amenorrhea.

In the normal, early fetus, the external layers of the embryo are known as the *trophoblast*. The trophoblast actively burrows into the uterine wall and is the means by which the fetus becomes embedded in the spongy decidua. A hydatidiform mole or trophoblastic disease can be regarded as an abnormal continuation of this locally aggressive behavior with unrestrained proliferation. Varying degrees of

hemorrhage and necrosis occur, and the overall appearances are usually characteristic (Fig. 5-23). However, a degenerating fibroid may occasionally give almost identical appearances. Because human gonadotropin is produced by the placenta, excessive amounts of this hormone are excreted in the maternal urine in trophoblastic disease. This can be measured by a quantitative UCG, in which the maternal urine is tested at increasing dilutions.

The prevalence of hydatidiform mole in the Caucasian race is approximately 1/2000. However, in the Phillipines the prevalence increases in 1/73 and in Taiwan 1/125. Thus, when ultrasound is practiced in areas with a high population of Orientals, hydatidiform moles are common.

Ovarian cysts commonly coexist with hydatidiform moles, due to the effects of increased hormone levels on the corpus luteum. This results in lutein cysts which are frequently bilateral. When typical appearances of a hydatidiform mole are seen within the uterus, combined with the presence of ovarian cysts in the adnexae, the sonographer will be more confident in making the diagnosis of hydatidiform mole.

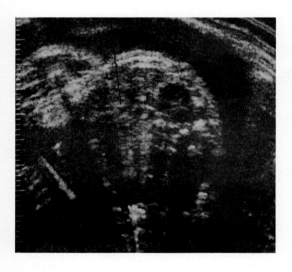

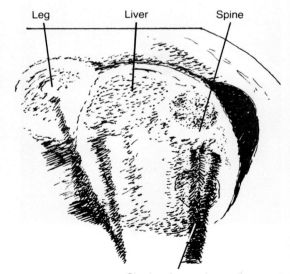

Fig. 5-19. Transverse scan through the mid-trunk showing the left and right kidneys separated by the spine. Note that there is shadowing from the spine. The fetal leg with shadowing from the femur is seen.

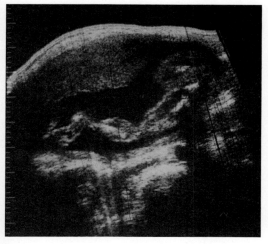

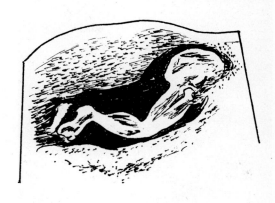

(A)

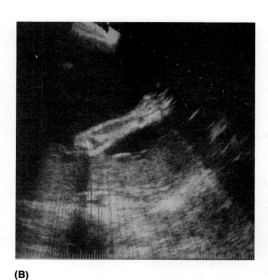

(B)

Fig. 5-20 **(A)** Details of the leg including the bony structure in the foot are seen. An anterior placenta is present. **(B)** Scan showing fetal arm with the digits well demonstrated. A posterior placenta is seen.

A tumor, especially a fibroid, is commonly seen coexisting with a fetus. The diagnosis is usually self-evident. However, a contraction ring may produce thickening of the myometrium which appears similar to a fibroid (Fig. 5-24). Painless uterine contractions occur throughout pregnancy. These were first described over a century ago by the British obstetrician Braxton Hicks, and are sometimes referred to as *Braxton Hicks contrac-*tions. These may last for 30 minutes at a time; the contracted uterine muscle may simulate a fibroid on ultrasound examination. They may be seen after amniocentesis when the needle puncture has induced a contraction. Any confusion can be clarified by rescanning the patient on a subsequent day when the thickened uterine wall should have relaxed and returned to normal. When the appearances persist a fibroid must be suspected.

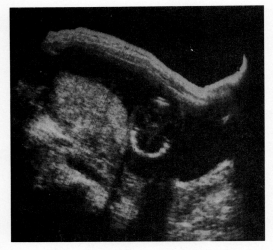
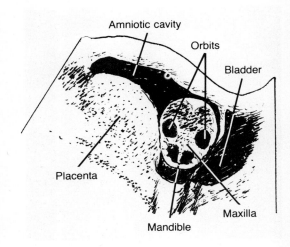

Fig. 5-21. Longitudinal scan showing details of the fetal head. The orbits, bony skeleton of the maxillary mandible can easily be demonstrated. A posterior placenta is seen.

Uterus Too Small For Dates or for the period of amenorrhea is most commonly caused by an incorrect date for the last menstrual period. This can be recognized in the first trimester by making an accurate crown-to-rump measurement. Another common cause is a missed abortion (blighted ovum). A number of definitions must be clarified at this point. A *threatened abortion* refers to vaginal bleeding in a pregnant patient from any cause. An *inevitable abortion* refers to vaginal bleeding with cramping uterine pain, implying that expulsion of the fetus is imminent. An *incomplete abortion* exists when there has been par-

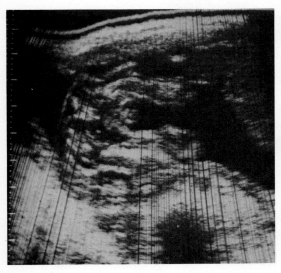
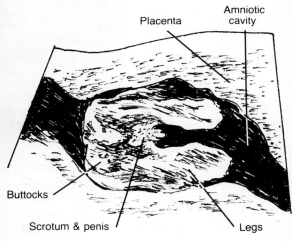

(A)

Fig. 5-22 **(A)** Transverse section to show legs and perineum of male fetus. Note that the scrotum and penis can be easily delineated. However, confusion may occur due to clitoral hypertrophy, or an incorrect tomogram. Thus, ultrasound can not be regarded as having more than a curiosity value for sexing infants.

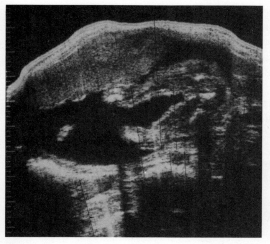

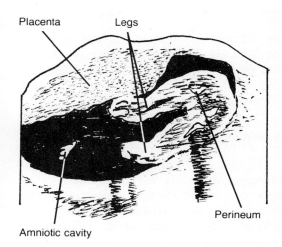

Placenta   Legs

Perineum

Amniotic cavity

(B)

Fig. 5-22 (Continued) **(B)** Legs and perineum of apparently female fetus, based on the absence of scrotum and penis.

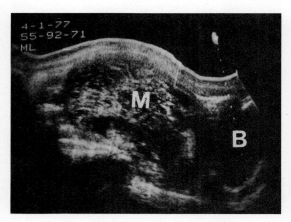

4-1-77
55-92-71
ML

M

B

Fig. 5-23. Longitudinal section through gravid uterus. The maternal bladder (B) is seen inferiorly. The uterine cavity is filled with placenta-like material (M) with many fluid-filled spaces due to necrosis and hemorrhage. These appearances are characteristic of a hydatidiform mole.

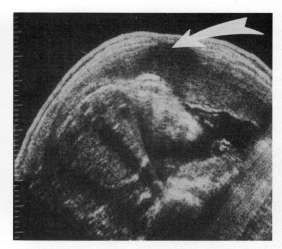

Fig. 5-24. A homogeneous mass is seen bulging the anterior uterine wall (arrowed). Although these appearances simulate those of a fibroid, such changes can be transient, representing uterine contraction rings.

tial evacuation of the fetus, but some products of conception, for example membranes or placenta, are retained within the uterus. A *complete abortion* occurs when there has been total evacuation of all products of conception from the uterus. And finally, a *missed abortion* occurs when there has been fetal death but no vaginal bleeding. This is sometimes referred to as a *blighted ovum*.

The ultrasound appearances of a missed abortion include an absent fetus, a collapsed or incomplete gestational sac or an apparently normal fetal contour, but without fetal activity. Doppler examination has been used to establish fetal activity, but it is easier to look for fetal heart movement either by putting an A-mode through the fetal thorax or by using real-time instrumentation.

Bleeding in the First Trimester

The differential diagnosis of bleeding in the first trimester includes a threatened, incomplete or inevitable abortion, a hydatidiform mole or other incidental pathology such as a fibroid or cervical polyp.

Abnormalities in Later Pregnancy

Uterus Too Large For Dates has a differential diagnosis which includes, as already considered, wrong menstrual dates, multiple gestation, hydatidiform mole, co-existent tumor or hydramnios (Fig. 5-25). *Hydramnios* refers to an excess of amniotic fluid, defined as a volume exceeding 1700 ml at 30 weeks, or 1000 ml at term. Using ultrasound, only qualitative estimations are available. Hydramnios is associated with at least four different conditions.

Fetal abnormality is associated with hydramnios. Fetal abnormality is present in 20 to 40 percent of fetuses with hydramnios. Most commonly the abnormality is that of the nervous system or gut. Hydrocephaly (Fig. 5-26), anencephaly (Fig. 5-27), spina bifida and meningomyelocele are all malformations of the central nervous system which are associated

with hydramnios. In addition, atresia of the gut, whether esophageal or duodenal, is associated with hydramnios, purportedly because of failure to absorb amniotic fluid after fetal swallowing.

Multiple gestation is also associated with hydramnios. This is a rarer cause of hydramnios in patients who already have one cause

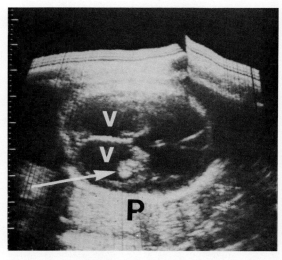

Fig. 5-26. Hydrocephaly. Transverse section through the fetal head to show markedly dilated ventricles (V); the choroid plexus (arrowed) is seen herniated into the lateral ventricles. The placenta (P) is seen posteriorly.

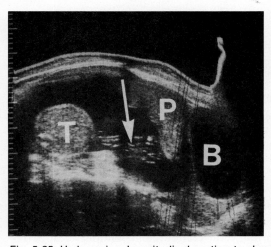

Fig. 5-25. Hydramnios. Longitudinal section to show maternal bladder (B), fetal trunk (T) in transverse lie, with an anterior, low lying placenta (P). Multiple loops of umbilical cord (arrowed) are seen. Notice that copious amniotic fluid is seen suggesting hydramnios.

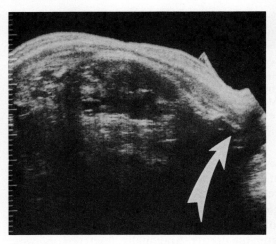

Fig. 5-27. Anencephaly. Longitudinal section through the fetus shows the vertebral column which when traced upwards shows no evidence of a normal fetal head (arrowed).

for a uterus too large for dates. Maternal diabetes is also a factor. This is commonly associated with hydramnios. Other conditions such as Rhesus incompatability, which will be discussed below are also associated with hydramnios.

Uterus Too Small For Dates or for the period of amenorrhea will have similar causes as those seen in the first trimester, including fetal death and incorrect dating. In addition, one must consider oligohydramnios and intrauterine growth retardation (IUGR). *Oligohydramnios* refers to a deficiency of amniotic fluid, specifically less than 400 ml in late pregnancy. This is associated with renal agenesis, reportedly because of the failure of the fetus to urinate. Due to this association, the kidneys should be carefully scanned if the patient is found to have oligohydramnios on ultrasound scanning.

Intrauterine Growth Retardation

There is a strong association between intrauterine growth retardation and oligohydramnios. Growth retardation is associated with "placental insufficiency." When growth is retarded, the biparietal diameter no longer remains an adequate parameter for estimation of

fetal maturity, since the growth of the fetal head is maintained at the expense of the body. Therefore, an early sign of inadequate nutrition is the failure of body growth. The circumference of the fetal trunk can be measured, and one can also look at the ratio between the size of the fetal head and the trunk. The placenta may be small and prematurely degenerating.

If IUGR is strongly suspected, biparietal diameters at 2 to 3 week intervals must be taken. The fetal trunk circumference may be measured on transverse scans using the level of the umbilical vein as a landmark. The area of the body is small compared with the size of the biparietal diameter in cases of IUGR (Fig. 5-28). In the 2nd trimester, the normal head circumference is greater than the abdominal circumference. Between 32 and 36 weeks, the body and head areas are equal, while after this, the body normally becomes larger than the head. Transverse scans are taken exactly at 90 degrees to the sagittal lie of the fetus to obtain the correct measurement.

Total intrauterine volume can be estimated as a further criterion of IUGR. For these calculations, the uterus is assumed to be an ellipse; the length, breadth and depth of the uterus must be measured from longitudinal

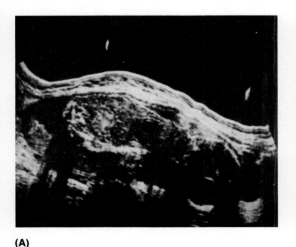

(A)

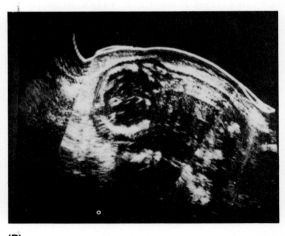

(B)

Fig. 5-28. Normal fetus **(A)** for comparison with intrauterine growth retardation (IUGR) **(B)**. Notice that the fetal trunk is small compared with the head. Placental insufficiency prevents growth of the body, but growth of the head is maintained. (Courtesy of John Hobbins, M.D.)

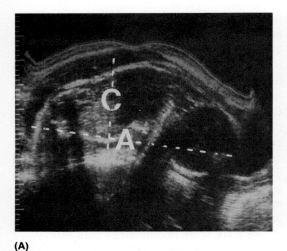

(A)

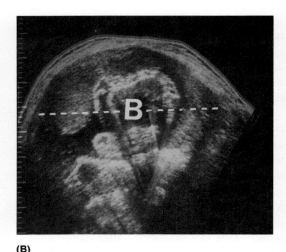

(B)

Fig. 5-29. Total intrauterine volume can be approximated assuming the uterus to be an elipse, of which the length (A), breadth (B) and the depth (C) are the axes.

and transverse scans (Fig. 5-29A and B). The total intrauterine volume (TIUV) is then calculated from the following formula:

$$V = \frac{4\pi}{3} \frac{\text{length [A]}}{2} \times \frac{\text{Breadth [B]}}{2} \times \frac{\text{Width [C]}}{2}$$

This can be condensed to V = 0.523 × ABC

TIUV increases rapidly near term when the change in biparietal diameter becomes minimal, and therefore unreliable. The earliest sign of IUGR is failure of TIUV to increase, resulting from failure of body growth, and decreased volume of amniotic fluid. If TIUV is 1.5 standard deviations or more below that expected from the biparietal diameter, the fetus is considered growth retarded (Fig. 5-30).

FETAL ABNORMALITIES

Hydrocephalus is produced by obstruction to the outflow of cerebrospinal fluid from the ventricular system of the brain (pp. 195–196). Hydrocephalus therefore results in dilatation of the ventricular system which allows its diagnosis. Because of the dilatation of the ventricular system, the head size is larger than

expected for the period of amenorrhea, and the head is disproportionately large for the trunk. This condition must therefore be differentiated from IUGR. The most useful criterion is visualization of a dilated ventricular system (Fig. 5-26). A secondary criterion is the common association of hydramnios with hydrocephaly, and oligohydramnios with IUGR.

Anencephaly refers to the failure of head development (Fig. 5-27). The earlier the diagnosis is made, the earlier a therapeutic abortion can be carried out. Not infrequently, however, these fetuses come to term undiagnosed, or are referred for ultrasound late in pregnancy to exclude a breech presentation. The absence of a normal fetal head makes the diagnosis evident. If these fetuses are born alive, they die shortly thereafter. Abnormalities of the central nervous system tend to run in families, and even in nationalities. For example, persons of Irish extraction have a higher incidence of central nervous system defects than those of Scandanavian extraction.

Other Central Nervous System Defects

These include a number of developmental malformations in the brain such as encephalocele or a porencephalic cyst. Spina bifida results from the failure of the vertebrae to fuse on the posterior aspect of the spinal cord. This failure of fusion may be minimal and result in no neurological deficit, and indeed may only be detectable on X-rays of the lumbar spine. Varying degrees of malfusion result in extension of the meninges through the defect which may produce a palpable mass in the lumbar region. This is termed *meningocele*. More severe degrees of malfusion result in the spinal cord and meninges being exposed. This is termed *meningomyelocele*. These patients are born paraplegic and will remain so throughout life. A serious consequence is the involvement of the urinary and rectal spincters, which will never function; the patient remains inconti-

nent throughout life. Unless treated carefully recurrent urinary tract infections occur and eventual death from renal failure occurs early in adult life.

In severe cases of spina bifida with exposure of the meninges and spinal cord to the environment the most serious complication is recurrent meningitis and eventual formation of hydrocephaly due to inflammatory adhesions which block the exits from the ventricular system in the brain. This can be detected and treated by various shunt operations, draining from the ventricular system in the brain either into the peritoneum or directly into the central veins.

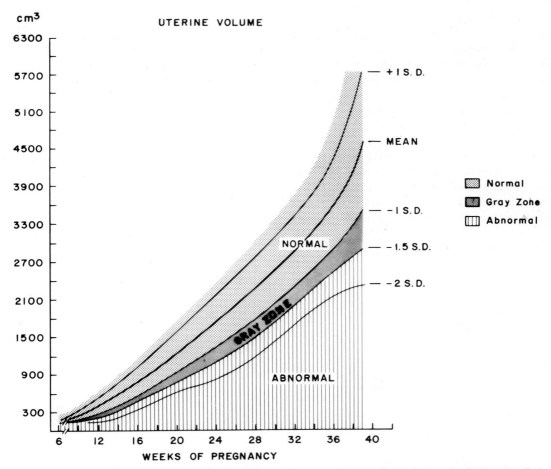

Fig. 5-30. Uterine volume: formula = length × width × thickness × 0.5233. (From Gohan, P., Berkowitz, R. L., and Hobbins, J. C.: Prediction of intrauterine growth retardation by determination of total intrauterine volume. Am. J. Obstet. Gynecol. 127:255, 1977).

Other Congenital Abnormalities

Without the aid of fetoscopy, only fairly gross abnormalities can be detected by ultrasound. Detectable abnormalities include polycystic kidneys, bilateral urinary tract obstruction resulting in hydronephrosis, renal agenesis (no kidney and no urine production), mesenteric and choledochal cysts, esophageal atresia (no fluid in gastric bubble) and duodenal atresia (hydramnios and a distended stomach).

Rhesus Incompatibility

Rhesus isoimmunization results when the mother who is rhesus (Rh) negative bears a rhesus positive child. Sensitized by the rhesus antigen, she forms antibodies which cross the placenta and cause hemolysis of the fetal red blood cells. The mildest form of the disease results in neonatal jaundice. However, with subsequent rhesus positive (Rh+) pregnancies and increasing exposure to the Rh factor, more antibody is produced and a severe form of isoimmunization occurs, resulting in edema and death of the fetus. This is known as hydrops fetalis.

Although interest originally focused on Rhesus isoimmunization as a major problem of blood group incompatability, immunization involving the ABO group is more common than that involving the Rhesus factor.

CONCLUSION

Ultrasound is now widely used to diagnose fetal presentation, age, viability and gross congenital anomalies, multiple gestation and placental position. More sophisticated techniques now allow the diagnosis of subtle congenital anomalies of the heart, central nervous system, urinary and alimentary tract. Serial measurements now permit monitoring of fetal growth and the diagnosis of intrauterine growth retardation.

SUGGESTED READING

Garvey MM, Govar ADT, Hodge C, Callander R: Obstetrics Illustrated, Second Edition. New York, Churchill Livingstone, 1974.

Hobbins JC, Winsberg F: Ultrasonography in Obstetrics and Gynecology. Baltimore, Williams and Wilkens Co., 1978.

Oxorn H, Foote WR: Human Labor and Birth. New York, Appleton-Century-Crofts, 1975.

Robinson HP: Gestation sac: volumes as determined by sonar in the first trimester of pregnancy. Br J Obstet Gynaecol 82:100, 1975.

Robinson HP: Sonar measurement of fetal crown-rump length as means of assessing maturity in first trimester of pregnancy. Br Med J 4:28, 1973.

Sabbagha RE, Turner JH, Rockette H, et al: Sonar BPD and fetal age. Definition of the relationship. Obstet Gynecol 43:7, 1974.

Taylor KJW: Atlas of Gray-scale Ultrasonography. New York, Churchill Livingstone, 1978.

6

Gynecology

CAROL A. TALMONT

INTRODUCTION

With the improved resolution of diagnostic ultrasound instrumentation, many invasive procedures used in the diagnosis and management of gynecologic patients may now be replaced. Presently ultrasound is used to diagnose complications in the first trimester of pregnancy; to identify and disclose the nature of any palpable masses, especially solid vs. cystic consistency; to locate intrauterine devices; and to evaluate patients with congenital anomalies of the genital tract.

Of these applications, those arising in the first trimester of pregnancy are by far the most important. During this time, no other imaging procedures or clinical examination can compete with the value of ultrasound in exposing the contents of the uterine cavity.

Anatomy

The internal sexual organs of the female comprise the vagina, uterus, Fallopian tubes, ovaries and the uterine ligaments including the broad ligaments. Of these, the uterus and ovaries are the organs optimally seen on ultrasound examination.

The Uterus is a thick-walled muscular organ situated between the urinary bladder anteriorly and the rectum posteriorly. It is a pear shaped organ and is approximately 7.5 cm (3″) long, 5 cm (2″) wide and 2.5 cm (1″) thick. In the mature female it weighs 30-40 grams. The uterine cavity joins the internal os, which continues down to the cervical cavity, the external os and the vagina. Upwards, the uterine cavity meets the Fallopian tubes, which spread out from the superior angles of

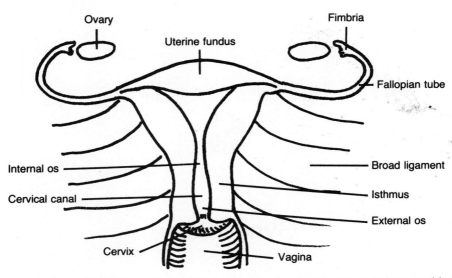

Fig. 6-1. Schema to illustrate normal anatomy. The uterus is a pear-shaped organ, continuous with the Fallopian tubes above. The distal end of the Fallopian tubes form a series of finger-like processes called the fimbria which are in direct contact with the ovaries. From the lateral edges of the uterus, a double fold of peritoneum called the broad ligament extends out towards the lateral wall of the pelvis. Inferiorly, the uterine cavity is continuous with the vagina through the cervical canal.

the uterus. They curve back on themselves and open in a series of finger-like projections known as the fimbria, which are in intimate contact with the ovaries. The ova are released into this fimbriated end of the Fallopian tube. Fertilization usually occurs within the Fallopian tube and the developing embryo (blastocyst) reaches the uterine cavity some three days after conception.

The anterior and posterior surfaces of the uterus are covered with a sheet of peritoneum which forms a double layer extending out across the pelvic cavity from the edge of the uterus. This is called the broad ligament of the uterus (Fig. 6-1). The Fallopian tube lies in the upper free edge of this broad ligament. The ovary is suspended on a short mesentery (mesovarium) from the posterior surface of the broad ligament.

The position of the uterus is variable, but in 90 percent of women it is anteverted and anteflexed, shown schematically in Figure 6-2. There is an angle of approximately 90 degrees between the axis of the vagina and the axis of the uterine cavity. This forward angulation of the uterus is called *anteversion*. In approximately 10 percent of women, the uterus is ret-

roverted, but this has essentially no pathologic significance. In addition to anteversion, the uterus is also slightly bent forward on itself, or *anteflexed*. Thus, in the normal female with an almost empty bladder, the uterus and the broad ligaments lie almost horizontal in the pelvic cavity. Obviously, if the bladder fills, the anteversion of the uterus becomes less marked, as the uterus is deflected posteriorly by the enlarging bladder. To understand the anatomy seen on ultrasound scanning, it is extremely important to know the peritoneal relations of the bladder. The peritoneum is a thin layer of tissue which lines the abdominal and pelvic cavities and defines the area which is occupied by the gut. The peritoneum is shown as a dotted line in Figure 6-2. Notice that the peritoneum sheaths the anterior aspect of the rectum and dips down to the most inferior part of the uterus, onto the highest part of the vagina (posterior fornix). The peritoneum is then reflected up over the posterior surface of the uterus. It covers the fundus of the uterus before passing onto the anterior surface of the bladder and up the anterior abdominal wall. This posterior peritoneal recess is known as the *recto-uterine pouch,* or *pouch*

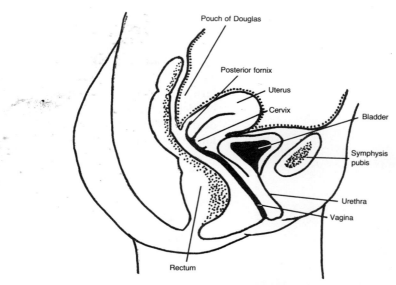

Fig. 6-2. Schema of sagittal scan through the female pelvis to show the normal position of the uterus which is anteverted and anteflexed. Note the fornices of the vagina surrounding the cervix and the pouch of Douglas (the rectouterine pouch) between the rectum and uterus. There is a further shallow peritoneal recess between the uterus and the bladder (utero-vesical pouch).

of *Douglas,* and is extremely important. Pathologically it is important because criminal abortions often involve laceration of the posterior vaginal wall with the introduction of bacteria into the peritoneal cavity, which may cause peritonitis and death. On ultrasound examination, the pouch of Douglas represents a recess which may become distended with ascites, pus, an ovarian cyst or loops of gut. Thus, material in the pouch of Douglas must be differentiated, and most importantly, material in the gut must not be confused with significant pelvic masses (pp. 91–92).

The Vagina is seen on ultrasound examination as a narrow tube ascending towards the cervix. The vagina is collapsed and appears as an anterior-posterior slit. It forms a cuff around the cervix, and each extension of the vagina around the cervix is known as a fornix. Thus, there are anterior, posterior and lateral fornices forming a rim around the cervix.

The Ovaries are attached to the posterior aspect of the broad ligament. The surface shows multiple scars which are the results of repeated ovulation. Each ovary is almond-shaped and is 3.5 cm long, 1.5 cm wide and 1.0 cm thick. The ovary has some degree of mobility since it is on a short mesentery (mesovarium). It is important to note that tumors and cysts derived from the ovary are also extremely mobile and may be adnexal in position, or present either anterior or posterior to the uterus.

SCANNING TECHNIQUE

The distended urinary bladder provides an acoustic window for ultrasound examination by deflecting the uterus posteriorly and displacing air-containing bowel out of the true pelvis.

Uterus Ultrasound may be used to evaluate the uterine size, the thickness of the myometrium and the size of the endometrial cavity. The sonographer can determine whether the bladder is sufficiently distended for examination of the uterus by scanning in the longitudinal plane. Scans are obtained in the parasagittal and sagittal planes every few millimeters, initially in the survey mode. Ultrasound is a tomographic technique and structures may be missed unless many tomograms are taken. Longitudinal, single-sector sweeps are performed to produce scans showing the following anatomy: distended bladder, uterus, cervix, and vagina (Fig. 6-3).

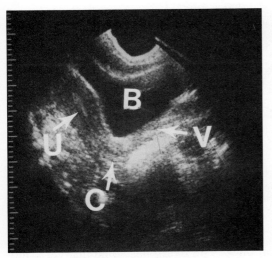

Fig. 6-3. Sagittal scan through the female pelvis demonstrating the urinary bladder (B) anteriorly. The uterus (U) is seen posterior to the bladder. The cervix (C) is seen at the junction of the uterus and vagina (V).

On longitudinal scans, the normal uterus appears as a pear-shaped organ which returns homogeneous, relatively low level echoes. It lies posterior to the distended urinary bladder. The endometrium presents an echogenic pattern within the uterine cavity. The cervix can be delineated at the point approximately 90 degrees between the axis of the vagina and the long axis of the uterus. (Fig. 6-4).

Transverse scans are obtained with a slight cephalad angulation of the transducer arm to take advantage of the distended bladder. Beginning at the symphysis pubis, in the continuous mode, the pelvis is surveyed in a superior direction. Transverse scans are recorded showing the body of the uterus, the broad ligaments and the ovaries. The three major pelvic sidewall muscles (iliopsoas, obturator internus and pubococcygeus) are visualized in the transverse plane (Fig. 6-5).

Ovaries The normal ovaries are delineated on either side of the uterus. They may be identified initially by scanning on the survey mode, on either side of the midline. On longitudinal sections, the transducer arm is angled laterally, which images the ovary separated from the fundus of the uterus.

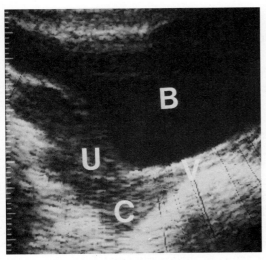

Fig. 6-4. Sagittal section showing magnified view of the cervix (C). The bladder (B) is anterior and the uterus (U) is seen posteriorly. The cervix projects into the upper extremity of the vagina (V).

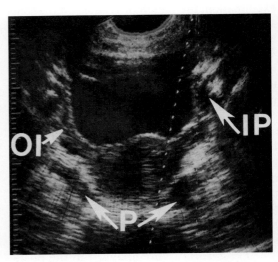

Fig. 6-5. Transverse section through the pelvis demonstrating the iliopsoas muscles (IP), obturator internus (OI) which lines the side wall of the pelvis and the pubococcygeus (P) which forms part of the pelvic diaphragm.

Transverse scans are performed on the survey mode, beginning at the midline superior to the symphysis pubis, and moving in short increments in a superior direction. The transducer is rocked by rotating it from the right pelvic side wall to the left (and vice versa) (Fig. 6-6). When both ovaries are located the continuous motion is stopped and the scan photographed. However, it is not always possible to locate both ovaries in the same transverse plane. Ovarian thickness, width and transverse inclination are evaluated on transverse scans. Normal ovaries can be visualized in approximately 90 percent of women during their reproductive years.

CLINICAL SYMPTOMS

Common gynecological complaints include those of abnormal vaginal discharge, abnormal menstrual cycle, pain or urinary symptoms, such as frequency. Pelvic inflammatory disease (PID) usually venereal in origin, presents with pain, vaginal discharge and often fever. In severe cases, constitutional symptoms such as nausea and vomiting may be reported. It is

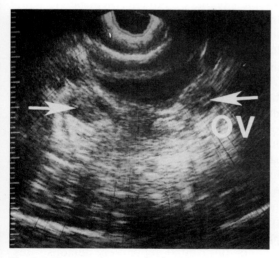

Fig. 6-6. Transverse scan obtained by sectoring through both adnexal regions from a midline placement of the transducer. The ovaries (arrowed, OV) are well seen, and are at the upper limits of normal in size, being 4 cm in maximal diameter.

important to establish the type of vaginal discharge the patient complains of. In PID, the discharge is classically purulent, that is, infected with organisms which make it either green or yellow in color. A white mucous discharge may be abnormal but is frequently within normal limits.

When considering abnormalities of the menstrual cycle the sonographer should be familiar with certain definitions. *Amenorrhea:* absence of menstruation. This may be primary amenorrhea in a female who has never menstruated, and is either physiological due to the young age of the female, or pathologic, perhaps due to a congenital abnormality. Secondary amenorrhea (acquired) is the cessation of menstruation after it has been established.

Dysmenorrhea: painful menstruation. This may also be primary or secondary. Primary dysmenorrhea often occurs for a short time in adolescence, in the absence of pathology. During adolescence, there is frequently failure to ovulate so that the menstrual cycles are painless. Primary dysmenorrhea commences with the onset of ovulatory menstrual cycles due to the secretion of progesterone which induces contractions of the uterus. This results in a midline, lower abdominal cramping, labor-type pain, which may be severe and accompanied by nausea, vomiting, headache and lower back pain.

Secondary dysmenorrhea has its onset later in life and is due to such pathological processes as endometriosis, chronic PID, ovarian tumors, fibroids or polyps. It is difficult to define when dysmenorrhea becomes pathologic but the following types of dysmenorrhea should be noted. Many normal women have an ill-localized but distressing pelvic congestion occurring for several days before the period and relieved with the onset of the period. Dysmenorrhea due to PID tends to mimic this congestion, but the symptoms become more severe. Endometriosis (see below) is another disease characterized by severe dysmenorrhea. However, the onset of pain is frequently one or two days before the onset of menstruation and persists or may become worse during the menstrual period. The ultrasonographer should be familiar with the occurrence of "Mittelschmerz" which is pain associated with ovulation and occurs exactly in the middle of the menstrual cycle, that is 14 days after the onset of the last menstrual period in women with 28 day cycles. It is probably due to intrafollicular pressure and possibly a small leak of blood or fluid as the ovum is discharged.

Polymenorrhea is abnormally frequent menstruation. *Menorrhagia* is excessively heavy menstruation. *Oligomenorrhea* is a condition of only slight menstrual loss.

Most abnormalities of the menstrual cycle in young patients have no organic cause which can be ascertained from clinical ultrasound examination. Such abnormalities are frequently called functional, which merely implies an absence of organic cause. However, with increasing age, abnormalities of the menstrual cycle secondary to some underlying disease become more common, so that the older patient must be energetically investigated to exclude serious but treatable disease.

CLINICAL APPLICATIONS

First Trimester Many of the problems in the first trimester of pregnancy have already been considered in Chapter 5. These may be summarized as follows: (1) early diagnosis of pregnancy; however, blood and urine tests are highly sensitive and much cheaper; (2) to assess fetal viability; (3) to determine fetal maturity (crown-rump measurements); (4) early diagnosis of multiple gestation; (5) to diagnose missed abortion, incomplete abortion and complete abortion; (6) to demonstrate incidental pelvic pathology such as a fibroid; (7) to exclude ectopic gestation; (8) to diagnose hydatidiform mole.

Ectopic Gestation A common problem in gynecological ultrasound scanning is the patient with a suspected ectopic pregnancy. *Ectopic gestation* refers to implantation of the embryo outside of the uterine cavity. Most commonly this occurs in the Fallopian tubes and is often secondary to previous PID which causes adhesions of the tubes and predisposes to ste-

rility or ectopic gestation. These patients usually present with pelvic pain and amenorrhea. The period of amenorrhea before the onset of symptoms depends on the site of implantation. If this is in the narrowest part of the Fallopian tubes (isthmus) it may present as early as six weeks amenorrhea because the embryo rapidly stretches the very narrow tube. Situated more laterally in the wider part of the Fallopian tube, ectopic pregnancies may not produce symptoms until 8 or 10 weeks. Approximately 5 percent of ectopics are found outside the Fallopian tubes, in the ovary or abdomen. An abdominal pregnancy is the only type of pregnancy which can reach term and is very difficult to diagnose by ultrasound. Obviously the ability to display the normal uterus in addition to the pregnancy immediately infers severe abnormality, which may include abdominal pregnancy or a pregnancy in one side of a double uterus (see below).

It must be stressed that ectopic gestation is an ultrasound and gynecologic emergency. Indeed, if undiagnosed, the tubes may rupture with catastrophic bleeding and possible maternal death. Ultrasound is by far the most satisfactory technique for demonstrating an early intrauterine gestation and thereby excluding an ectopic. Because the symptoms of possible ectopic pregnancy (amenorrhea, pelvic pain) are very common and nonspecific, a large number of patients are screened for ectopic gestation by ultrasound. These patients should all have pregnancy tests (beta sub unit, or UCG). If the pregnancy tests are positive, then the gestational sac must be identified by ultrasound before the patient can be allowed to leave the hospital. If an intrauterine gestational sac is identified by ultrasound, the patient can leave, but if ultrasound fails to demonstrate the intrauterine gestational sac in the presence of a positive pregnancy test, the patient must be subjected to further investigations including laparoscopy or even laparotomy. In a small number of these patients, ultrasound definitively demonstrates an extrauterine pregnancy and the patient proceeds to laparotomy. (Fig. 6-7).

The actual incidence of ectopic gestation varies in different series from one in 3,000, to

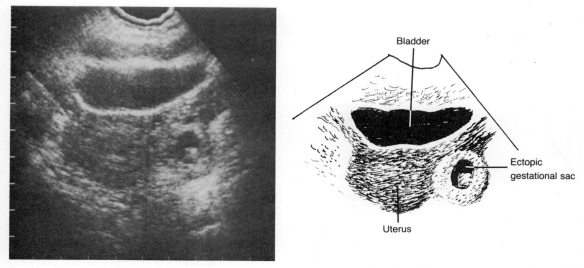

Fig. 6-7. Transverse scan to show an ectopic pregnancy. The uterus contains a moderate decidual reaction but a definite gestational sac is seen in the left adnexal position. Real-time examination or M-mode may reveal fetal viability.

one in 125, depending largely upon the incidence of veneral disease in the population. However, the fear of ectopic pregnancy results in two to three referrals per day at this institution. Many of these patients have had a culdocentesis before or after being referred for ultrasound examination. This procedure involves the aspiration of fluid from the cul de sac (pouch of Douglas) via the fornix of the vagina. If blood is aspirated which does not clot, it is considered to be free fluid in the peritoneum, or could be from a leaking ectopic pregnancy. Although this is a time honored method for the diagnosis of ectopic pregnancy, the overall accuracy is only approximately 75 percent, so that confidence in it can not be high.

Hydatidiform Mole Hydatidiform mole is also a serious problem that may occur in early pregnancy. On clinical examination, the uterus is usually larger than expected from the menstrual history. The most common symptoms associated with hydatidiform mole are vaginal bleeding and excessive vomiting in early pregnancy. Ultrasound examination shows many fluid filled spaces within placenta-like material (pp. 73–77).

Clinical Applications in the Nonpregnant Patient

Simple Cysts are the most common adnexal masses. Most are ovarian in origin and are well-defined, echo-free areas, with smooth borders, a strong posterior wall and good through transmission of the ultrasound beam. (Fig. 6-8). Septa may be present. Ovarian cysts may be located anywhere in the pelvis, anterior, posterior, superior or lateral to the uterus, and ultrasound has proved to be an excellent modality for assessing their location and size. If the cyst measures over 6 cm in diameter there is a possibility of torsion and rupture. Subsequent examinations are carried out to follow these cysts, which may undergo spontaneous absorption. Such follow-up ultrasound examinations have prevented surgery for numerous patients. Generally, a high frequency transducer is used for good delineation of cyst walls.

Dermoid Cysts (Cystic Teratoma) are curious tumors derived from the ovary, and should be regarded as a disorganized attempt to produce a fetus. The tumors have elements of all the primitive body tissues (endoderm, ectoderm and mesoderm). Thus, skin is present which grows hair and secretes sebaceous material. Thyroid glandular tissue may be present, as well as bone and even teeth. The presence of pelvic teeth has been used as a classic means for diagnosing dermoid cysts.

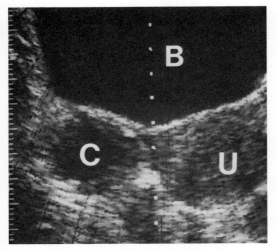

Fig. 6-8. Transverse section to show an adnexal ovarian cyst. The bladder (B) is seen anteriorly and the uterus (U) posteriorly. In the right adnexal position there is a rather thick walled, small ovarian cyst (C).

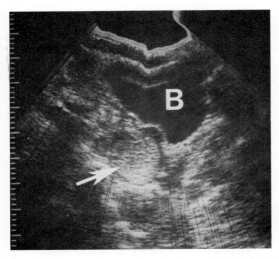

Fig. 6-9. Paramedian section to show a dermoid cyst. The bladder (B) is seen anteriorly. In the adnexal position, posterior to the bladder, an echogenic mass is seen (arrowed). Such echogenic masses must be differentiated from bowel contents, but are consistent with dermoid cysts.

However, in our experience over the past three years, most dermoid cysts we have diagnosed have not contained such bony elements and have been invisible on radiography.

The patient suspected of having a dermoid cyst may experience dull unilateral pain. A dermoid usually appears on ultrasound examination as a mass with areas of increased density which may shadow (Fig. 6-9).

Leiomyomas or Fibroids   appear on ultrasound as homogeneous, solid, space-occupying masses within the uterus (Fig. 6-10). However, when undergoing degeneration or necrosis, areas of sonolucency may appear. Fibroids may undergo calcification and be highly echogenic, with distal shadowing (Fig. 6-11). They cause irregular borders and enlargement of the uterus and may occur singly or in numbers. A fibroid may be attached to the uterus only by a stalk and such a pedunculated fibroid simulates a solid adnexal mass such as an ovarian cancer.

Endometriosis   occurs classically in nullipara over the age of 30. It is a disease characterized by endometrial tissue (lining of the uterus) situated in ectopic sites such as the peritoneum, adnexae, ovaries and broad ligament. Bleeding from these ectopic sites occurs with menstruation. The presence of blood in the peritoneal cavity produces a dense, fibrotic reaction which may result in hard, adnexal masses of fibrosis almost indistinguishable from cancers. However, most frequently these masses appear as fluid-filled areas which may simulate abscesses. They may contain blood and give sufficient internal echoes to simulate a solid tumor. Since changed blood becomes brown these are often referred to as *"chocolate" cysts* or *endometriomas* (Fig. 6-12).

A similar pathological process has been described which involves primarily the myometrium and this is known as *adenomyosis*. In our experience at this institution, endometriosis and adenomyosis frequently coexist, so that when fluid-filled lakes are seen scattered throughout the myometrium, the possibility of adenomyosis and endometriosis should be considered.

Pelvic Inflammatory Disease (PID)   can be evaluated with ultrasound, although the

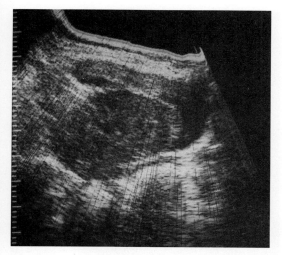
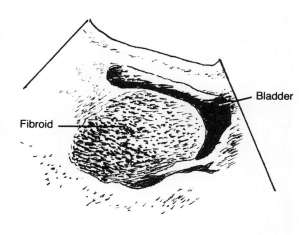

Fig. 6-10. Parasagittal scan showing a large, fibroid uterus.

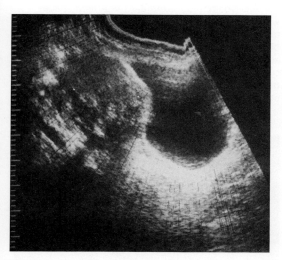
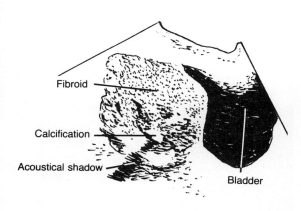

Fig. 6-11. Sagittal scan showing a large, fibroid uterus. High level punctate echoes within this uterus with distal shadowing are characteristic of calcified fibroids.

scans may show nonspecific changes identical to those seen in endometriosis. The classical lesion of PID is a tubo-ovarian abscess. This is a complex mass, partially solid and partially cystic, seen in the adnexal position or posterior to the uterus in the pouch of Douglas (Fig. 6-13).

Ovarian Carcinoma occurs in women 50 to 60 years of age and is frequently advanced before diagnosis. Ultrasound, therefore, could be important as a method for early detection of ovarian cancer. It is apparent either as a solid enlargement of the ovary or as a partially cystic, partially solid mass, as seen in a cystadenocarcinoma (Fig. 6-14A and B). Ovarian carcinomas have irregular walls, and the condition must be suspected in any postmenopausal patient with a solid adnexal mass. Both benign and malignant ovarian tumors may cause ascites, and this fluid is noted both in the pelvis and in Morison's pouch. Ovarian tumors, or tumors arising from the uterus may

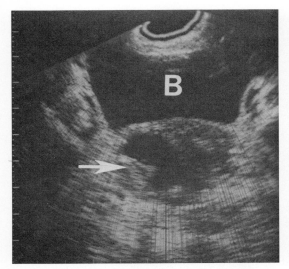

Fig. 6-12. Transverse section. The bladder (B) is seen anteriorly. In the right adnexal position there is a complex, but mainly fluid-filled mass (arrowed). These appearances are consistent with a pelvic abscess, chocolate cysts, or a complex ovarian cyst. Surgery revealed an endometrioma (chocolate cyst).

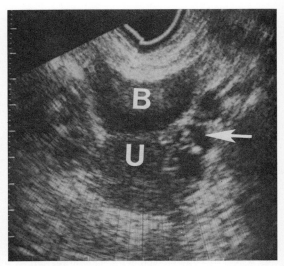

Fig. 6-13. Transverse scan showing the bladder (B) anteriorly, and the uterus (U) posteriorly. In the left adnexal position are irregular fluid-filled spaces which could be due to pelvic inflammatory disease or endometriosis. Bowel contents must be differentiated by real-time examination or repeat scanning. In this patient the clinical signs and symptoms were consistent with pelvic inflammatory disease; these scans also show a tubo-ovarian abscess.

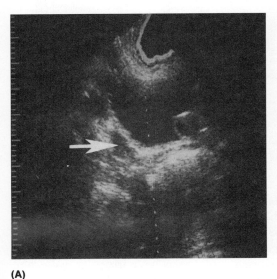

(A)

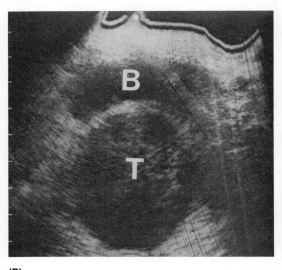

(B)

Fig. 6-14. (A) Sagittal scan of a 70-year-old patient showing small, post-menopausal, atrophic uterus (arrowed). Note that a Foley catheter balloon is seen in the bladder. (B) Scan of pelvis of post-menopausal woman. The bladder (B) is seen anteriorly. A large, predominantly solid tumor (T) is seen posterior to the bladder. It is often not possible to tell whether such a tumor is uterine or ovarian in origin. However, benign tumors such as fibroids do not increase in size after menopause, so that such pelvic tumors occuring in post-menopausal women are usually malignant.

extend towards the lateral wall of the pelvis and involve the ureters, thereby producing hydronephrosis. Because of this association, whenever a mass is seen in the pelvis of a middle-aged woman, the upper abdomen should be scanned to rule out hydronephrosis or evidence of distant metastases to the liver, peritoneum or omentum.

Intrauterine Devices Ultrasound is useful in the management of the patient with an intrauterine contraceptive device (IUD). In assessing the intrauterine location of an IUD, 100 percent accuracy can be obtained. Both metallic and polyethylene devices are visualized. However, the technique is of limited value if the IUD perforates the uterus, since it is difficult to differentiate the echoes of an IUD from the irregular, multiple echoes of fecal material in the bowel.

The Copper-7 (Fig. 6-15) and Lippes loop appear as highly reflective linear echoes within the endometrial cavity. A Lippes loop is identified in the sagittal plane as five dashes (Fig. 6-16). The Copper-T or -7 is identified on ultrasound as a vertical line on the longitudinal scans (Fig. 6-17). The transverse scans demonstrate the upper portion of the device as a horizontal line (Fig. 6-18). The presence of an IUD with an intrauterine gestation may be identified early by ultrasound.

Congenital Abnormalities Ultrasound is increasingly being used to investigate internal genitalia of young patients with intersex states (Fig. 6-19A and B). In most of these patients a satisfactory physical examination is difficult or impossible to obtain, and at this instituion the use of ultrasound is preferred. The presence of an infantile uterus can be identified, and in patients on hormone therapy, the growth of the uterus and ovaries with therapy can be monitored by repeated ultrasound examinations.

A bicornuate uterus is one common congenital anomaly which should be considered in detail. To comprehend the origin of this anomaly, it is necessary to consider briefly the embryology of the uterus and Fallopian tubes. The Fallopian tubes, uterus and upper two-

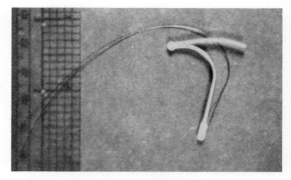

Fig. 6-15. Copper-7 intrauterine device.

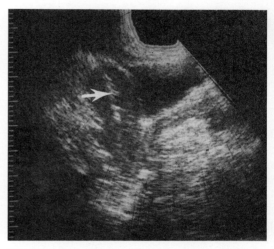

Fig. 6-16. Sagittal section showing an intrauterine Lippes loop (arrowed).

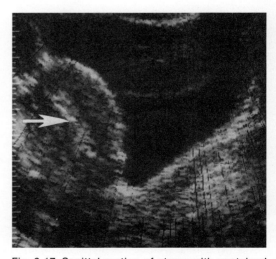

Fig. 6-17. Sagittal section of uterus with contained Copper-7 intrauterine device (arrowed).

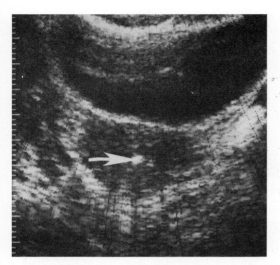

Fig. 6-18. Transverse pelvic scan of uterus containing a Copper-7 device (arrowed). Note that there is distal shadowing beyond the IUD.

thirds of the vagina are derived from tubes called the Mullerian ducts. In normal development, these two ducts, which lie parallel to each other, fuse from the lower end up. Fusion followed by canalization results in the hollow vagina being continuous with the uterus, while the upper ends remain unfused as the Fallopi-

an tubes. However, all degrees of malfusion can occur and these are shown schematically in Figure 6-20 A to C. A septate uterus (A) shows a double uterine cavity resulting from malfusion. The presence of this septum may not be apparent from clinical examination or at surgery. A more severe degree of malfusion is seen in the bicornuate uterus (B). This has the greatest importance in the pregnant patient, since the condition may predispose to recurrent abortion. The condition can also lead to some perplexing clinical problems. We have seen patients who have undergone two therapeutic abortions, presumably because the wrong uterus was scraped. In late pregnancy, ultrasound appearances of a bicornuate uterus with a pregnancy in one cornu may be indistinguishable from those of an abdominal pregnancy. For all these reasons, a bicornuate uterus is an important entity with which the sonographer should be familiar. Complete failure of fusion gives a double uterus (C), a double cervix and double vagina. This is known as a didelphic uterus with a double vagina.

CONCLUSION

Ultrasound may now be regarded as an essen-

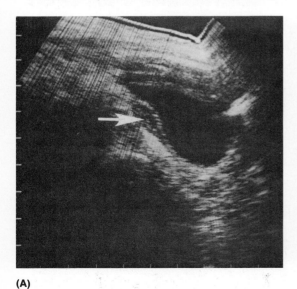

(A)

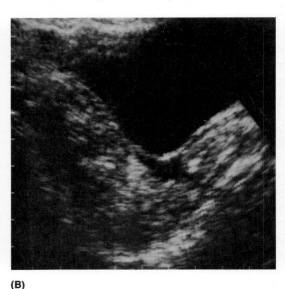

(B)

Fig. 6-19. (A) Normal pre-pubertal uterus (arrowed). Notice that the cervix is approximately as long as the body of the uterus. (B) Uterine agenesis. Genetically this patient was a male, but had normal female external genitalia.

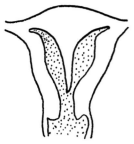
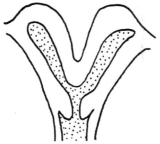
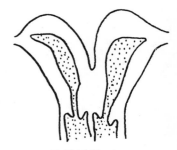

A Septate uterus   B Bicornuate uterus   C Didelphic uterus

Fig. 6-20. Schema to show results of nonfusion of the Müllerian tube derivatives. **(A)** Minimal malfusion results in a septate uterus which may not be apparent on physical examination. **(B)** Moderate degree of malfusion of the uterus resulting in a bicornuate uterus. A pregnancy may occur in one cornuum only. **(C)** Complete malfusion of the uterus so that a double uterus is present (didelphic uterus). More extensive degrees of malfusion of the Müllerian duct system give rise to double cervix and double vagina.

tial imaging modality for diagnostic use in the first trimester of pregnancy. It has now replaced IVP and barium enema as the initial imaging technique for assessing the presence and type of pelvic mass. Since the advent of gray-scale ultrasound, gynecologic diagnosis by ultrasound has become much more useful, and certain abnormalities, such as congenital anomalies, ovarian cystadenomas, carcinoma, dermoid cysts, tubo-ovarian abscesses and adenomyosis present highly characteristic findings. Although some diseases present rather nonspecific findings, the results of ultrasound examination may be helpful when taken in conjunction with the clinical history.

SUGGESTED READING

Sample WF, Lippe BM, Gyepes MT: Gray-scale ultrasonography of the normal female pelvis. Radiology 125: 477-483, 1977.

Taylor KJW: Gynecology. In: Atlas of Gray-Scale Ultrasonography, Edinburgh, Churchill Livingstone, 1978.

Walsh JW, Rosenfield AT, Jaffe CC, Schwartz PE, Simeone J, Dembner AG, Taylor KJW: Prospective comparison of ultrasound and computerized tomography in the evaluation of gynecologic pelvic masses. AJR 131:955-960, 1978.

Walsh JW, Taylor KJW, Rosenfield AT: Gray-scale ultrasonography in the diagnosis of endomentriosis and adenomyosis. AJR 132:87-90, 1979.

7

Liver

KENNETH J. W. TAYLOR
PAULA JACOBSON

INTRODUCTION

The liver is the largest organ in the body, but much of it lies deep to the lower ribs, so that the normal sized organ is difficult to examine clinically. It is however, the most frequent site for metastatic disease, and for diffuse changes such as cirrhosis, both of which are common in the United States.

The liver and spleen can be imaged by isotopic techniques using ^{99m}technetium (Tc) labelled colloids. Colloidal particles are taken up by the cells of the reticuloendothelial system. This system comprises the lymphoid tissue and nodes, the spleen and Kuppfer cells of the liver. These tissues become labelled with radioactive ^{99m}Tc because they take up the colloid particles by phagocytosis. Radioactivity in the liver and spleen is then imaged by a gamma camera. When a space-occupying mass replaces the normal tissue which con-

tains Kuppfer cells, a cold area is apparent on the scans. This technique has a number of advantages.

1) The method is widely available and well standardized.

2) It can be used in the obese patient and those with extensive dressings.

3) ^{99m}Tc is a radiopharmaceutical which gives a low dose of ionizing radiation and is relatively economic.

4) The examination does not require much technician skill.

5) It provides an overview of the entire liver.

However, isotopic scans do have three disadvantages.

1) There is relatively poor resolution, at best 2 cm in vivo.

2) The examination is nonspecific, in that areas of diminished uptake may be due to any space-occupying lesion, whether it is a benign

cyst, abscess, vascular malformation or malignant tumor.

3) And there is frequent confusion between anatomical variation in the contour of the liver and defects due to significant pathology, especially in the region of the porta hepatis, the right renal fossa and the gallbladder fossa.

Because of these problems, ultrasound examination is extremely valuable both to add specificity by differentiating between cyst and tumor and to clarify the equivocal scan by demonstrating normal anatomy or a pathological space-occupying mass.

Anatomy of the Liver

The liver comprises right and left lobes, with two small subdivisions of the left lobe called the quadrate and caudate lobes. The shape of the liver is partially determined by the imprint of the structures surrounding it. The superior surface is snug against the diaphragm. Posterior to the right lobe of the liver is the right kidney and adrenal gland. Anteriorly and laterally, the liver is in contact with the anterior and lateral abdominal wall. The liver tapers towards the left. The under surface of the liver (visceral surface) slopes upward from the anterior border to the posterior border and is in contact with the stomach, colon, duodenum and gallbladder. On this visceral surface of the liver is the porta hepatis, which is the entrance for the hepatic arteries, the portal vein and the exit for the left and right hepatic (bile) ducts. The posterior surface of the liver has a variable relationship to the inferior vena cava which may be posterior to it, or deeply imbedded in it. The hepatic vein, the main left, right and middle hepatic veins drain directly into the inferior vena cava. The porta hepatis is a transverse fissure which divides the quadrate lobe anteriorly from the caudate lobe posteriorly. This differentiation is clearly apparent on ultrasound scanning.

The relation of the structures entering and leaving the liver at and below the porta hepatis must be understood. The portal vein ascends from behind the neck of the pancreas where it is formed, passing to the right with varying degrees of obliquity to reach the porta hepatis. Just before the porta hepatis, the portal vein divides into left and right portal branches, and these again can be seen on ultrasound examination. In its passage towards the porta hepatis, the portal vein is accompanied by two important structures which are located anterior to it. The common bile duct is anterior to the portal vein and to the right, while the hepatic artery is anterior to the portal vein and to the left. These three structures are wrapped in a double-fold of mesentery which runs from the duodenum to the porta hepatis. This peritoneum is known as the lesser omentum or gastrohepatic ligament. These three structures lie immediately anterior to the inferior vena cava although separated from it by peritoneum and a slit (the epiploic foramen), which is the entrance to the lesser sac behind the stomach. This relationship must be recalled in parasagittal scans which show the inferior vena cava in longitudinal section. Anterior, lies the portal vein with the common bile duct anterior. On real-time ultrasound equipment, the hepatic artery can easily be seen pulsating in this position.

Blood Supply of the Liver

The liver is an unusual organ in that it has a double blood supply: the hepatic artery and the portal vein. Approximately 20 percent of the blood supply is from the hepatic artery, the remainder from the portal vein. The portal venous system is important for normal metabolism, since it consists of a double system of capillaries. The arteries supplying the gut break down into a capillary bed where digested material is absorbed. The veins draining from the intestine (inferior mesenteric and superior mesenteric) join the splenic vein to form the portal vein. The portal vein then breaks up into a second capillary bed within the liver. This allows metabolites and end-products of digestion within the gut to be metabolized by the liver. This function of the liver produces one of the common symptoms of liver failure—encephalopathy, i.e., signs and symptoms of mental derangement due to absorption of materials such as ammonia which reach the systemic circulation instead of being metabolized and detoxicated in the liver.

Physiology of the Liver

Any detailed consideration of the physiology of the liver is clearly beyond the scope of this book, and the reader is referred to textbooks already available. In this section we deal only superficially with some of the symptoms and signs of patients with liver disease who present for ultrasound examination. These functions include the metabolism of bile pigments and transformation of water insoluble bilirubin-protein complex into water soluble bilirubin glucuronide (pp. 113 – 114). In the presence of impaired hepatic function, the bilirubin level rises in the serum. This bilirubin is water insoluble, the so-called indirect reactive.

Another function is the synthesis of certain proteins including albumin and fibrinogin. Albumin is an important serum protein which is responsible for the plasma osmotic pressure. When the serum albumin is low, fluid is not reabsorbed from the tissue spaces, resulting in edema and ascites. Ascites is very common in end-stage cirrhosis. Low serum albumin is noted on tests for serum proteins, and there is usually compensatory increase in serum globulin levels. Fibrinogen is a protein which is important in blood clotting, so that abnormal bleeding tends to occur in advanced liver disease.

Protein metabolism and formation of urea from ammonia are also functions of the liver. An elevated level of serum ammonia is a contributing cause of encephalopathy which accompanies liver failure.

Fat metabolism occurs in the liver. Many important fats are synthesized in the liver, and bile salts are necessary for fat absorption. Bile salts are important detergents which permit the absorption of fat by rendering fat particles water soluble. In liver failure, fat soluble vitamins A and K are not absorbed. Deficiency of vitamin K leads to abnormal bleeding, so that patients with severe liver disease are poor surgical candidates.

Carbohydrate metabolism is yet another function. The liver stores glycogen which is a stored form of carbohydrate and, under the influence of insulin, controls the serum levels of glucose.

The metabolism of drugs and hormones must also be considered. The sex hormones are inactivated and metabolized in the liver, and in the presence of impaired liver function, these sex hormones accumulate. Appreciable levels of estrogens are present in the male, produced by the adrenal cortex. High levels of estrogens in the presence of hepatic failure produces abnormal breast development (gynecomastia), testicular atrophy and small vascular malformations (spider nevi).

The liver contains cells of the reticuloendothelial system, known as Kuppfer cells. These are responsible for ingestion of foreign particles and are involved with the immune response. The capacity of these liver cells to absorb injected foreign particles is the basis of the isotope imaging technique involving intravenous injection of ^{99m}Tc colloids, previously discussed. However, because of the highly nonspecific nature of the isotope scan, the specificity of ultrasound liver examination is essential.

This section has briefly reviewed some of the major functions of the liver to explain the symptoms and signs of liver failure. The liver is clearly responsible for a magnitude of different functions and contains a large number of enzymes which can be used as markers of liver disease. When the liver is injured, such as in hepatitis, cell damage causes the release of these enzymes into the blood. Important enzymes include lactic dehydrogenase (LDH), serum glutamic oxaloacetic transaminase (SGOT), serum glutamic pyruvic transaminase (SGPT) and 5-nucleotidase. Few of these enzymes are peculiar to the liver: for example, LDH is also elevated after myocardial infarction. There are subtle differences in the structures of these enzymes from different organs; these organ-specific enzymes are known as isoenzymes. Although myocardial LDH can be differentiated from the liver LDH isoenzyme, at the present time this differentiation is too expensive to be a practical procedure. The secretion of alkaline phosphatase into the bile from the walls of the biliary tree is considered on p. 114. Again, a different isoenzyme of alkaline phosphatase may be elevated in bone disease. Thus elevation of the serum levels of these enzymes may be indicators of liver disease but are not unique to liver damage. However, these enzyme values should be extracted from the patient's medical record and noted on the requisition for ultrasound examination, since this will guide the interpreting physician to careful examination of the liver parenchyma in a search for diffuse or focal disease.

SCANNING TECHNIQUE

To scan the liver, the patient initially lies in the supine position. Mineral oil is copiously applied to the abdominal surface except in patients who are unable to bathe, and then a water soluble coupling agent is used. Right upper quadrant masses may be palpated during this procedure, and the correlation between ultrasonographic appearances and a palpated mass should be carried out by the physician. A history of alcohol abuse or known primary carcinoma are pertinent parts of the history. For patients with known metastatic disease, history of treatment with chemotherapy is important as this may affect the appearances of the metastases.

If the patient has had a ^{99m}Tc colloid liver/spleen scan, the results should be noted on the requisition so that interpretation of the ultrasound scans is carried out in conjunction with the isotope scans. It has been demonstrated that equivocal liver/spleen scans can be accurately assessed by directed ultrasound scans. The area of defect on the liver/spleen scan should be known to the sonographer and special attention given to the corresponding area of the liver.

A proper TGC curve is essential to visualize small, subtle lesions. The A-scan through the right lobe of the liver (Fig. 7-1A) should be examined. Set correctly, internal echoes from the liver parenchyma should be approximately $1/3$ to $1/2$ the size of the echo returning from the diaphragm. Even on the A-scan diaphragmat-

ic movement can be confirmed by asking the patient to inspire deeply while observing the A-scan. Improper TGC setting (Fig. 7-1B) gives an uneven distribution of echoes throughout the liver parenchyma. Excessive anterior gain overwrites the superficial parts of the liver (Fig. 7-2) with insufficient trans-

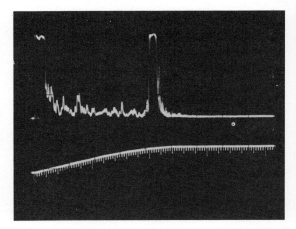

(A)

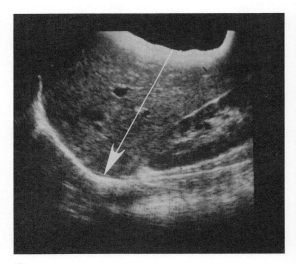

(B)

Fig. 7-1. **(A)** The normal A-scan (above) and the correct TGC curve (below) for a beam placed across the liver towards the diaphragm. Notice that the intrahepatic echoes are relatively small compared with the diaphragm and are of similar amplitude throughout the liver. **(B)** B-scan showing the liver and right kidney with correct TGC. Diaphragm is arrowed.

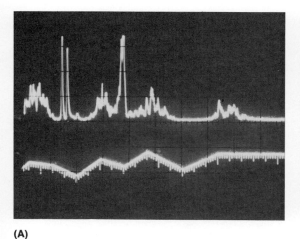 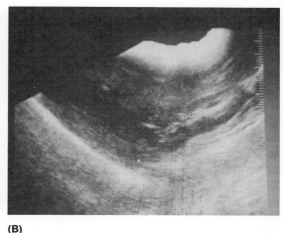

(A)   **(B)**

Fig. 7-2. **(A)** Iregular A-scan through the liver, due to incorrect TGC setting seen on the lower trace. TGC through a homogeneous organ such as the liver should be virtually a straight line. (Note that this is logarithmic scale since attenuation is logarithmic.) **(B)** B-scan corresponding to the TGC setting seen in **(A)**.

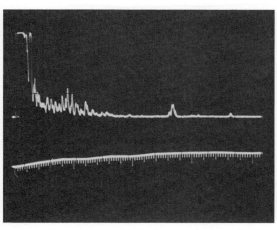 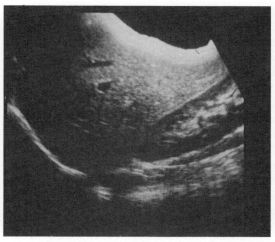

(A)   **(B)**

Fig. 7-3. **(A)** Inadequate TGC resulting in insufficient amplification of the distant echoes. Notice that the echo from the diaphragm is very small. **(B)** B-scan corresponding to the TGC seen in **(A)**. Notice that the deeper parts of the liver are inadequately imaged due to inadequate gain.

mission to the posterior region. Figures 7-3 and 7-4 show excessive distal gain, so that the anterior surface of the liver is inadequately written and the posterior is overwritten.

Scanning is commenced with sagittal sections taken through the liver. The equipment may be set on continuous motion so that multiple scans can be taken to the left and right of the midline to visualize the entire left and right lobes. The entire liver parenchyma must be written, from the diaphragm to the inferior border, with the patient holding deep inspiration. If gas in the gut obscures the liver, one may have the patient blow out the abdomen, thereby pushing the gas inferior to the liver. While scanning the left lobe of the liver, the sonographer should identify the aorta, the ce-

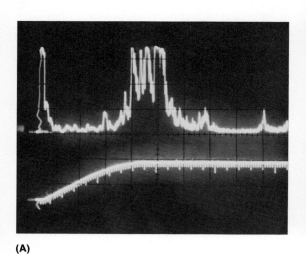

(A)

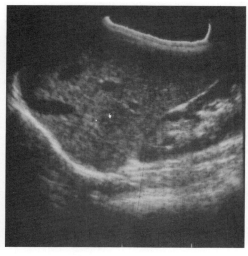

(B)

Fig. 7-4. **(A)** Inadequate TGC on the anterior aspect of the liver. **(B)** B-scan corresponding to the inadequate anterior gain shown in **(A)**.

liac trunk, superior mesenteric artery (SMA), superior mesenteric vein (SMV), left hepatic vein and left branch of the portal vein (Figs. 7-5A and B). Scanning further towards the right, the inferior vena cava (IVC), middle hepatic vein and portal vein can be seen. The caudate lobe of the liver can be visualized superior to the portal vein (Fig. 7-6). Continuing to the right, the right kidney can be seen on the posterior aspect of the liver. The right hepatic vein and the right branch of the portal vein are also seen.

A highly effective view of the liver is obtained from a sector scan performed perpendicular to the right costal margin (Fig. 7-6 and 7-7). The sonographer should again begin at the far edge of the left lobe with the patient holding deep inspiration, and continue through the porta hepatis into the right lobe, making short angled single sector scans.

Transverse scans are commenced just inferior to the xiphisternum, using sector scans which arch under the right and left costal margins and the lateral edges of the liver. The right, middle and left hepatic veins can be seen draining into the inferior vena cava at this level. Scanning inferiorly, the celiac trunk, portal vein, splenic vein, SMV, SMA, IVC,

aorta and renal arteries and veins can be visualized (Fig. 7-8). Scans should be continued sequentially and inferiorly past the right kidney to the very tip of the liver.

These transverse or oblique scans are important for investigating the left and right lobes of the liver simultaneously. Occasionally one lobe of the liver will be totally replaced by tumor and on parasagittal scanning a huge tumor may be missed; since the major difference between metastatic disease and normal liver parenchyma is a small difference in the amplitude of the returned echoes, a large tumor area may be misinterpreted as insufficient overall gain. Increasing the gain may cause a tumor to simulate normal parenchyma. Scans which visualize both lobes of the liver may allow better comparison between normal and abnormal tissue.

To view the most lateral parts of the liver adequately and to exclude a peripheral tumor or subphrenic abscess, intercostal sector scans are made. Multiple scans are carried out in every available intercostal space on the anterior and lateral aspects of the abdominal cavity (Fig. 7-9). When there is excessive gas, or body habitus makes optimal visualization of the entire liver difficult, left side down decubi-

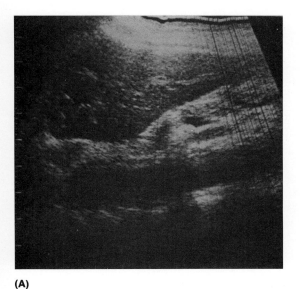

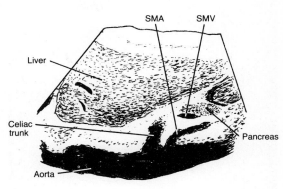

(A)

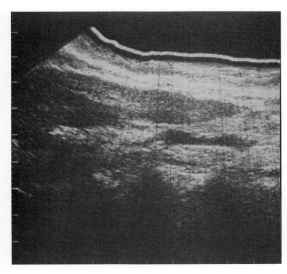

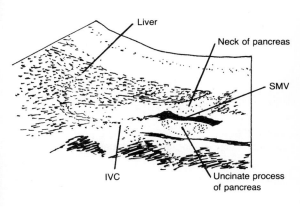

(B)

Fig. 7-5. **(A)** Longitudinal section in the plane of the aorta. The celiac and superior mesenteric (SMA) arteries can be seen. The most cephalad portion of the superior mesenteric vein (SMV) is seen immediately deep to the body of the pancreas. **(B)** Longitudinal section in the plane of the inferior vena cava (IVC). The superior mesenteric vein (SMV) is well seen. Superficial to the SMV is the densely reflective neck of the pancreas, while deep to it is the uncinate process.

tus postion may be helpful in obtaining the necessary scans. These can be carried out in the transverse, coronal or oblique planes.

When a defect is suspected on one scan or plane, the same defect must be shown in an-other projection before it can be considered valid. A defect which appears to be on the in-ferior border of the liver may be due to stom-ach, pancreas, gallbladder or colon. The pa-tient may be given a glass of water to change

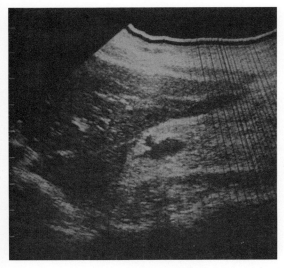
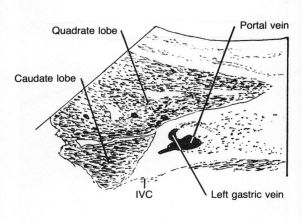

Fig. 7-6. Longitudinal section in the plane of the inferior vena cava (IVC). The portal vein and branches are seen. Note that the liver in this position is divided into the caudate lobe posteriorly and quadrate lobe anteriorly by a sheet of fibrous tissue.

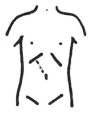

Fig. 7-7. Schema to show scanning plane perpendicular to the right costal margin.

the appearance of the stomach and thus allow its recognition. Alternatively the patient's position may be changed to either the upright or decubitus. This movement causes movement of the viscera, such as the colon, away from the liver edge.

Diffuse Abnormalities of the Liver

The sonographer should be alert to diffuse changes in the liver parenchyma. Fatty infiltration is common and produces an increased amplitude of echoes throughout the liver, often with dilated veins (Fig. 7-10). Fatty infiltration can be produced secondary to congestive cardiac failure, obesity, but most commonly is due to alcoholic liver disease. Indeed, the

most common diffuse parenchymal liver disease in the USA is alcoholic liver disease. In an ultrasound/histological correlation carried out at this institution, we found that ultrasound was capable of detecting 2+ fat or fibrosis (on a scale of 1 to 4), but not capable of differentiating between them.

Typically the cirrhotic liver consists of dense white echoes anteriorly, but with markedly increased attenuation which leads to inadequate penetration to the posterior surface (Fig. 7-11). These findings are obviously obtained with a normal TGC setting. The TGC can be modified by reducing the anterior gain and increasing the overall gain to reduce the amplitude of the echoes to uniformity across the liver substance. Even then, the parenchymal echo amplitude will be found to be similar to that emanating from the diaphragm instead of $\frac{1}{3}$ of that amplitude. These findings indicate intrahepatic fibrosis due to a number of various causes, but most commonly associated with alcoholic liver disease. Because of the obstruction of the portal venous radicles as they ramify into the liver substance, obstruction of the portal venous inflow occurs. The result of the portal vein obstruction is the development of an enlarged, tortuous portal vein and superior mesenteric

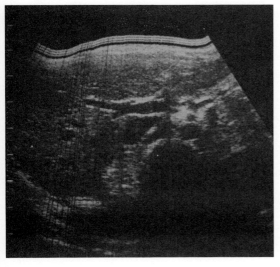

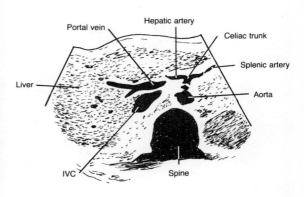

(A)

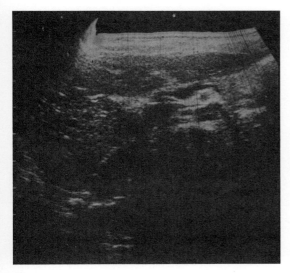

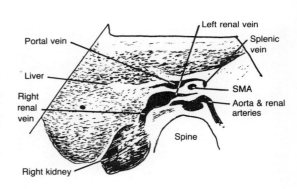

(B)

Fig. 7-8. **(A)** Transverse scan showing the major vessels. The celiac trunk divides into the hepatic and splenic arteries. The right branch of the portal vein passes into the liver substance before dividing into anterior and posterior branches. **(B)** Transverse scan showing important vasculature of the upper abdomen. The left and right renal veins are seen draining into the inferior vena cava (IVC). The splenic vein enters the superior mesenteric vein to form the portal vein. The superior mesenteric artery is seen anterior to the aorta, and the renal arteries are seen.

vein. The back pressure effects produce progressive congestive splenomegaly. In patients with suspected portal hypertension, the spleen should be scanned for splenomegaly. The enlarged spleen can be examined with the patient supine. Less obvious splenomegaly requires scanning techniques detailed in Chapter 12 (pp. 158–160). Scans performed in the oblique

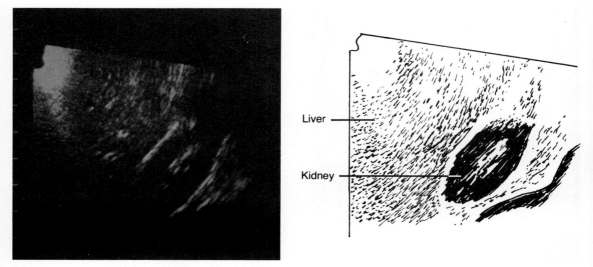

Fig. 7-9. Transverse sector scan to show liver and right kidney. This is a valuable technique to demonstrate imited views of the liver when it is high under the costal margin and subcostal scanning is impossible.

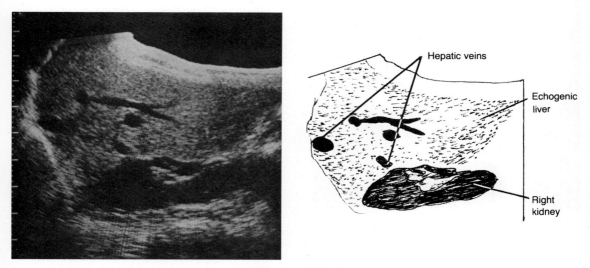

Fig. 7-10. Longitudinal scan through the liver showing enlargement with venous dilatation. Appearances are suggestive of chronic venous congestion and consistency suggests fatty infiltration as a result of longstanding congestion.

intercostal axis of the spleen should measure 10 cm or less. In patients with portal hypertension and congestive splenomegaly, the char- acteristic internal consistency is more echo- genic than normal spleen and the longitudinal axis measures 12 to 18 cm.

Focal Defects of the Liver

Cysts Incidental cysts of the liver are not uncommon and are usually of no pathological significance. They are more frequent in the right lobe of the liver than in the left, and in women more than men. Often these patients are referred because of a positive isotope scan, although they do not clinically appear to have metastatic disease of the liver. A liver cyst is shown in Figure 7-12. The sonographer should establish the size and position of the cyst, note the presence of any partial or complete septa within it, and note the presence of any debris. Typically, benign incidental cysts are virtually completely echo free. The A-scan through the cystic lesion should be photographed in addition to the B-scan. The A-scan should be almost completely flat with exaggerated echoes distal to the lesion. This distal enhancement is due to the addition of TGC which allows for tissue attenuation; however, tissue attenuation does not occur as the ultrasound beam passes through the fluid contents of the cyst. Thus the echoes distal to the cystic lesion have received excess compensation for attenuation. Liver cysts are often septated but

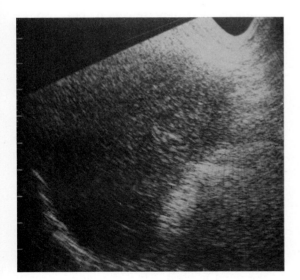

Fig. 7-11. Longitudinal scans through the right lobe of the liver showing abnormal consistency with increased echo amplitude and increased attenuation. Appearances are suggestive of cirrhosis.

usually have regular walls. The presence of debris within a cyst raises the possibility that this could be a necrotic tumor and not a simple cyst.

In obese patients the A-scan through a cystic area may not be completely flat, possibly due to multiple reverberations through adipose tissue. In such patients, an A-scan through fluid located within that patient's body should be taken for comparison with the A-scan taken through the respective cystic lesion. Either the contents of the gallbladder or the urinary bladder are suitable fluid collections for A-mode comparison. If the A-mode through the suspected cystic lesion is similar or lower in amplitude than the echoes obtained from the bladder or gallbladder contents, the cystic nature of the lesion is confirmed.

Liver cysts frequently co-exist with polycystic kidney disease, and in these patients, the cystic lesions are frequently extremely irregular in contour and the cystic renal masses are virtually indistinguishable from the cystic masses in the liver.

Cystic lesions within the liver may occasionally result from necrosis within a malignant tumor, and this is more commonly seen in patients who have been energetically treated. Typically these patients have debris within the cystic lesion, there is an irregularity of the walls of the cyst and there is a solid component within the wall of the cyst. In these patients, the entire liver should be carefully scanned to search for solid tumor deposits in addition to the partially or completely necrotic ones which tend to focus the attention. Again, the A-mode through the lesion should be photographed and compared with A-modes through fluid filled viscera in the obese patient.

Complex Lesions Complex lesions are focal masses which contain both fluid and solid components. Such lesions include many inflammatory masses forming abscesses as well as partially necrotic malignant tumors. Often differentiation between these two types of pathology is not possible from the ultrasound scans alone, but is relatively easy when the pertinent history is also considered.

The peritoneum around the liver dictates to some extent the anatomical localization of fluid collections which gravitate to the liver. When a patient is in the supine position, the area between the right lobe of the liver and the right kidney (Morison's pouch) is the lowest part of the abdominal cavity, so that any pus from the abdomen tends to drain into that subphrenic space and may form an abscess there. Other common sites for abscess formation (p. 149) are the subhepatic spaces in which abscesses are frequently seen associated with gallbladder disease or surgery, intrahepatic abscesses or left subphrenic abscesses.

Typically an abscess has a fluid filled center with irregular thick walls, and there are often high level echoes around the abscess cavity (Fig. 7-13). Differentiation between hematoma, necrotic tumor, abscess cavity or cavernous hemangioma may not be possible on ultrasound appearances alone, although the clinical history aids considerably in this interpretation.

Solid Lesions *Primary Liver Tumors.* Benign tumors of the liver are rare although there are reports of increasing numbers of hepatic adenomas in young patients who have been on contraceptive pills. These lesions, however, are so rare that our experience to date has

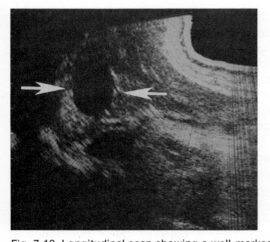

Fig. 7-12. Longitudinal scan showing a well-marked defect (arrowed) in the upper portion of the liver. This lesion is virtually anechoic and appearances are consistent with a simple liver cyst.

only included two such lesions, which have been highly reflective.

Malignant primary tumors of the liver include the hepatoma and cholangiocarcinoma. A hepatoma is extremely variable in ultrasonic appearances. In our experience at this institution, 25 percent of echogenic liver tumors proved to be hepatomas. However, a complete spectrum of ultrasonic appearances are seen, including an almost completely necrotic malignant cyst. These tumors tend to supervene in patients with established cirrhosis, when small tumors may be confused with regenerating nodules. However, generally regenerating nodules are not differentiated by ultrasound, so that a focal lesion seen within a cirrhotic liver must be carefully documented and the presence of a hepatoma must be suspected.

Cholangiocarcinomas are primary liver tumors arising from the bile ducts. They may be located at the junction of the left and right hepatic ducts and present very early with obstructive jaundice. This type of tumor is known as a Klatskin tumor.

Metastatic Disease to the Liver. The ultrasound appearances of metastases show wide variation in reports from different centers. This may be partly explicable in terms of differences in patient selection, but also we believe is partially dependent on video format and the quality of ultrasound images. For example, when bistable machines were used to detect liver metastases, albeit extremely unsuccessfully, echogenic metastases were the only types of tumors which were recognized. This was because the normal parenchyma was not displayed, therefore defects of it were not detected. With increasing ability to display the parenchyma faithfully, defects which were only slightly different in echo amplitude from the normal tissue become apparent. It has been our experience that echogenic metastases are more obvious if the white background is used, while relatively echo-free metastases appear more obvious if a black background is used. Thus the video formats used at different centers may affect the overall accuracy with which these types of tumors are detected.

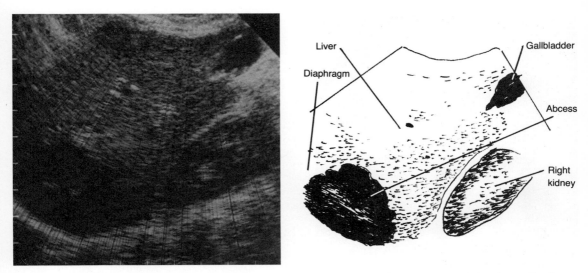

Fig. 7-13. Longitudinal scan through the right lobe of the liver. Note that there is a large defect immediately beneath the right hemidiaphragm in a patient with fever and elevated white blood count. This is consistent with a large subdiaphragmatic abscess.

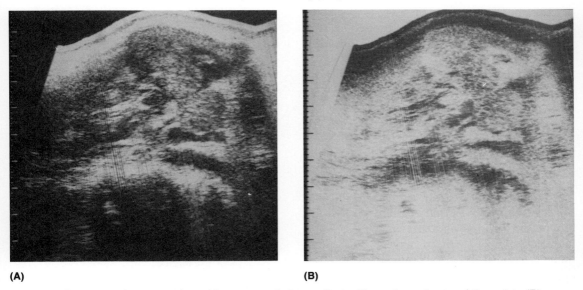

(A)   **(B)**

Fig. 7-14. **(A)** Echogenic metastasis and hepatomegaly in a patient with a primary tumor of the colon. **(B)** Echogenic metastases are also well seen using a white background. However, for subtle metastases of lower amplitude than the normal parenchyma the use of a white background can make identification extremely difficult. For this reason we prefer the use of a black background.

Metastatic disease to the liver may produce focal zones of decreased echogenicity, increased echogenicity or mixed lesions. Although some authors deny any correlation between tumor type and ultrasound appearances, this is not the general experience. Many ultrasonologists report that echogenic metastases (Fig. 7-14A and B) are most frequently found from primary tumors in the colon. Thus if the patient presents with multiple

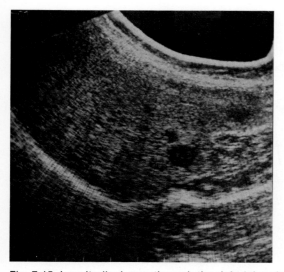 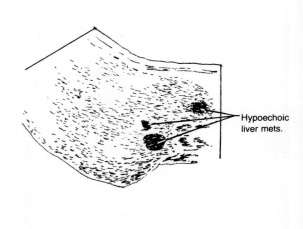

Hypoechoic
liver mets.

Fig. 7-15. Longitudinal scan through the right lobe of the liver showing three small focal defects which return slightly lower level echoes than the normal parenchyma. Note that the smallest tumor discretely imaged is approximately 1 cm in diameter, and this size is beyond the resolution of gamma cameras using technetium sulphur colloid.

echogenic lesions scattered throughout the liver, the possibility of a colonic primary should be investigated with barium studies. We have also noted that a substantial number of these echogenic lesions proved to be hepatomas.

Approximately one-third of liver metastases return echoes which are lower than those of the surrounding normal liver parenchyma (Fig. 7-15). For example, in patients with carcinoma of the breast, the majority have relatively echo free liver metastases. Multiple scans over a period of time may show dimunition or slow increase in the size of a metastatic lesion with the possible development of central necrosis. Thus, there may be definite changes in size and ultrasonic characteristics with time and treatment.

CONCLUSION

In conclusion, ultrasound can be used very successfully for diagnosing both focal and diffuse disease of the liver. Although isotopic visualization of the liver and spleen is a valuable screening technique in which the entire organ is imaged, ultrasound adds specificity.

Thus the real value of ultrasound of the liver is in differentiating anatomical variation from significant pathology in an equivocal liver/spleen scan, in differentiating cold areas on liver/spleen scanning into cyst, abscess or tumor, in detecting small lesions beyond the resolution of isotope scanning and in investigating the jaundiced patient.

SUGGESTED READING

Leevy CM, Popper H, Sherlock S: Diseases of the Liver and Biliary Tract. Standardization of Nomenclature, Diagnostic Criteria and Diagnostic Methodology. DHEW pub. no.76-725, 1976.

Sherlock S: Diseases of the Liver and Biliary System. 5th Ed. Oxford, Blackwell Scientific, 1975.

White TT, Sarles H, Benhamon J-P: Liver, Bile Ducts and Pancreas. New York, Grune & Stratton, 1977.

Taylor KJW (ed): Diagnostic Ultrasound in Gastrointestinal Disease. New York, Churchill Livingstone, 1979.

Taylor KJW, Carpenter DA, McCready VR, Hill CR: Grey-scale ultrasound imaging. The anatomy and pathology of the liver. Radiology 119:415-423, 1976.

Taylor KJW, Rosenfield AT: Grey-scale ultrasonography in the differential diagnosis of obstructive jaundice. Arch Surg 112:820-825, 1977.

Taylor KJW, Sullivan D. Rosenfield AT, Gottschalk A: Grey-scale ultrasound and isotope scanning: Complementary techniques for imaging the liver. AJR 128:277-281, 1977.

8

Biliary System

PAULA JACOBSON
KENNETH J. W. TAYLOR

INTRODUCTION

Ultrasound has revolutionized the investigation of the jaundiced patient, since it permits the immediate, noninvasive visualization of the biliary tree, both in the normal and dilated states. For the diagnosis of gallbladder disease, oral cholecystography remains the elective screening procedure, but ultrasound has achieved wide application for the diagnosis of gallbladder disease in patients who are unsuited for oral cholecystography. These include patients with nausea, vomiting, diarrhea, jaundice and those with acute cholecystitis. The accuracy of the procedure is comparable to that of oral cholecystography.

Anatomy and Physiology

The biliary system is responsible for the secretion and excretion of bile. It looks like a tree,

in which all the branches are within the liver, and only the two main stems and the trunk lie outside the liver. These stems are the left and right hepatic ducts and the trunk is the common bile duct. The common bile duct opens, usually with the pancreatic duct, into the descending (second part) duodenum. Figure 8-1A shows this schematically, while Figure 8-1B shows a cast from an actual biliary tree. Note that the branches divide frequently, so that any slice through the liver would reveal multiple short sections which branch frequently. This is apparent on ultrasound and helps to distinguish the biliary tree from the branches of the portal venous system. The divisions of the hepatic ducts are the biliary ductules, and the subdivision continues down to the finest twigs, which form the biliary canaliculi. These are microscopic structures. Thus, bile produced by the liver cells is passed into the finest radicles of the biliary tree, gradually passing

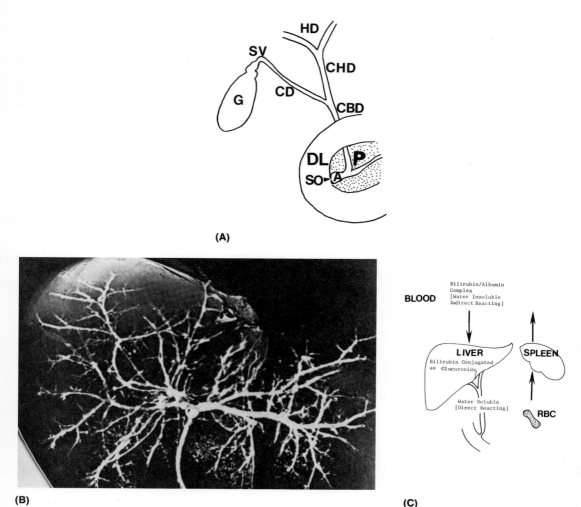

(A)

(B)   **(C)**

Fig. 8-1. **(A)** Schema to show the anatomy of the portal system. The left and right lobes of the liver are drained by the left and right hepatic ducts (HD) respectively. The hepatic ducts combine to form the common hepatic duct (CHD), which is joined by the cystic duct (CD) to form the common bile duct (CBD). The junction of the cystic duct with the common bile duct is variable. The common bile duct passes posterior to the duodenum where it is related to the anterior aspect of the portal vein and passes on the deep surface of the head of the pancreas (P). The arrangement of the duct is variable, but it is frequently joined by the pancreatic in a dilated area known as the ampulla (A), before opening into the duodenum. This opening into the duodenum is guarded by the sphincter of Oddi (SO). The pancreatic head is encompassed by the duodenal loop (DL). The gallbladder should be regarded as a diverticulum from the main biliary system. If bile does not pass down into the duodenum because of contraction of the sphincter of Oddi, it refluxes up the cystic duct into the gallbladder (G). There bile is concentrated by the absorption of water. A valvular arrangement is found in the neck of the gallbladder, known as the spiral valve (SV). **(B)** Perfusion study of the bilary tree, demonstrating early bifurcation into multiple vessels of similar caliber (Reprinted from Ultrasound in Medicine, ed. White DN, 4:125-134, 1978. With kind permission of Plenum Press). **(C)** Schema to show metabolism of bilirubin. Old red cells are broken down in the spleen or other parts of the reticuloendothelial system with the production of bilirubin. This forms a complex with albumin in which it is transported in the blood. In this protein complex the bilirubin is water insoluble and is indirectly reacting. In the liver the albumin is removed and the bilirubin is conjugated with glucuronic acid. The bilirubin is now water soluble and directly reacting. It is then excreted in the biliary tree as shown in Figure 1A. It should be apparent that excess breakdown of red cells or liver failure largely result in an excess of the water insoluble (indirectly reacting) bilirubin, while an obstruction to the biliary tree results in an increase in water soluble (direct reacting) bilirubin.

into bigger and bigger branches and finally draining into the left or right hepatic ducts from the respective lobes of the liver and into the common bile duct. The entrance of the common bile duct and pancreatic duct into the duodenum is guarded by the sphincter of Oddi. A dilated segment immediately before this sphincter is known as the ampulla of Vater and a tumor of the ampulla or a stone impacted in it, produces obstruction of the entire biliary tree.

The gallbladder is a diverticulum from the biliary tree which acts as a temporary reservoir for the storage of bile between meals. Bile is probably secreted almost continuously and drains down the biliary tree. If the sphincter of Oddi is open, it drains into the duodenum, but when the sphincter is closed, bile refluxes up the cystic duct from the common bile duct and distends the gallbladder.

The gallbladder is variable in shape, size and position. It is usually situated on the inferior surface of the liver, lateral to the inferior vena cava and portal vein and anterior to the right kidney. However, it may be embedded in the liver (intrahepatic) or suspended on a mesentery, in which case it is even more variable in position (wandering gallbladder). In our experience the normal gallbladder can measure up to 12 cm in length. An obstructed gallbladder may be smaller than this but is usually spherical in contour, rather than the elongated, pear-shape of the unobstructed gallbladder. An intricate arrangement of the mucosa is found at the neck of the gallbladder as it passes into the cystic duct. These are the valves of Heister and are of importance in ultrasound, since they may cast a shadow, probably due to collagen within them and may simulate a stone impacted in the neck of the gallbladder.

The function of the bile is partially excretory and partially secretory. Bile contains both bile pigments and bile salts (sodium taurocholate and glycocholate). These bile pigments are important for the proper absorption of fats, since they act essentially as detergents, rendering fat water-soluble and capable of being absorbed. In the absence of bile salts, there is failure of fat absorption with the subsequent excretion of excess fat in the stools and, in particular, the loss of important fat-soluble

materials, including vitamins A, D and K. Bile pigments (biliverdin and bilirubin) are also excreted in the bile and these are essentially end-products of the breakdown of red blood cells. Bile salts are largely reabsorbed in the colon and re-excreted by the liver, to form what is called "enterohepatic circulation". However, some bile pigments are excreted in the feces and are responsible for their characteristic color. In the absence of bile, the stools become white and fatty due to excessive excretion of unabsorbed fat.

Required Laboratory Data

It is most important for the interpreting physician to note the direct and total bilirubin. The bilirubin may be elevated due to three reasons. Excess bilirubin may be produced by the breakdown of red blood cells, for example, in hemolytic diseases. Liver disease may be present, so that bilirubin accumulates because it is not metabolized and excreted by the liver. Or there may be obstruction to the biliary tree which prevents excretion.

Causes of jaundice can therefore be subdivided into prehepatic, hepatic and posthepatic or obstructive causes. These causes of jaundice can be differentiated to some extent by estimating the amount of serum bilirubin which is direct acting, as opposed to that which is indirect acting. The metabolism of bilirubin must be briefly considered to understand the significance of this (Fig. 8-1C). The reticulo-endothelial cells are responsible for the ultimate breakdown of red blood cells and release bilirubin from the hemoglobin within the red blood cells. This bilirubin is combined immediately with plasma proteins and transported as a complex with albumin. This is insoluble in water and is the indirect reacting bilirubin. The protein-bound bilirubin is further metabolised in the liver cells. Bilirubin is removed from the protein and conjugated with glucuronic acid to form a glucuronide which is water soluble. It is in this form that bilirubin is excreted into the bile and is direct reacting. The total bilirubin is the sum of that which is water soluble (direct acting) and water insoluble (indirectly reactive). Thus, if most of the elevated bilirubin is direct reacting, this implies that the bilirubin has been metabolized by the liver, and that the cause of jaundice is a post-hepatic obstruction. If most of the bilirubin is in the indirect form, then it has not been metabolized by the liver, and either excessive bilirubin has been formed, overwhelming the metabolizing capability of the liver temporarily, or the liver function itself is compromised.

A further laboratory test to determine the level of biliary obstruction is the estimation of the serum-alkaline phosphatase. Normal levels are less than 80 iu (one must be certain that international units (iu) are being used rather than the old King Armstrong units). Alkaline phosphatase is produced by the walls of the biliary tree and excreted in the bile. If there is obstruction to the excretion of bile, alkaline phosphatase refluxes back into the blood stream, and the alkaline photophatase level rises significantly. However, alkaline phosphatase is not specific to the liver, and levels of a similar isoenzyme are also raised in certain bone diseases.

Many other enzymes may be elevated when there is associated liver disease; two important ones are lactic acid dehydrogenase (LDH) and serum glutamic-oxaloacetic transaminase (SGOT). (See p. 99).

Tests of pancreatic function include serum amylase and serum lipase. Both of these are transiently elevated in acute pancreatitis, and persistant elevation may also occur in the presence of a pseudocyst.

The white blood cell count is an important laboratory test in patients with suspected inflammatory conditions of the biliary tract. These include acute cholecystitis, empyema of the gallbladder and cholangitis. An empyema of the gallbladder occurs when the gallbladder is filled with pus. This is a serious condition requiring early surgery. Cholangitis is an inflammatory condition involving the bile ducts themselves, and obstruction with bile stasis predisposes to infection.

TECHNIQUE

Results of the clinical data, when available, should be extracted from the patient's record and noted on the ultrasound requisition to aid the physician in subsequent interpretation. These data are also important for follow-up purposes. The sonographer should palpate the right upper quadrant, noting the presence of any obvious masses which require identification by ultrasound scanning, as for example, a hydrops of the gallbladder. During this procedure, any pain on palpation should be noted. If the patient complains of pain, its anatomic location, character, relation to meals, in particular fatty meals, should be established. The presence of obvious jaundice is apparent especially from observation of the sclerae. It should be established either from the patient's chart or direct questioning and other tests which the patient has undergone for subsequent correlation.

To scan the gallbladder and biliary tree, the sonographer sets the TGC similar to that used for examining the liver (pp. 100–101). Using these settings, sections are taken in the parasagittal plane, through the inferior vena cava and portal vein. The sonographer must search the liver parenchyma for any signs of dilatation of the intrahepatic biliary ducts. Anterior to the portal vein, the common bile duct is sought, with special reference to the lower portion of it, deep to the head of the pancreas. Next, sections are taken in the midline, left of the plane of the inferior vena cava, identifying the superior mesenteric vein and artery and the aorta. Sections are then taken towards the right, inspecting the liver parenchyma and the normal intrahepatic biliary ductules. These vessel walls are usually virtually in apposition, with less than 2 mm between them. Separation of 2 mm or more represents an abnormally dilated biliary tree. In sections taken to the right, the gallbladder usually becomes apparent, lying anterior to the right kidney. Depending upon the depth of the gallbladder, the frequency of the transducer may be changed to 3.5 MHz, with a short or medium internal focus. In some of the latest machines, a frequency as high as 5 MHz can be used with ease, while in very obese patients, frequencies of 2.5 MHz must be used to penetrate the layer of fat and minimize the scatter

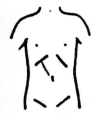

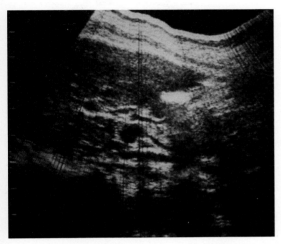

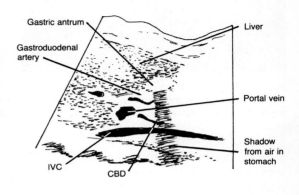

Fig. 8-2. Parasagittal scan 2 cm to the right of the midline showing the inferior vena cava (IVC) posterior to the portal vein. Note that the head of the pancreas is sandwiched between the gastroduodenal artery and the common bile duct.

from the subcutaneous fat. Multiple sagittal sections through the neck and the body of the gallbladder are taken to determine the size, shape and position of the gallbladder while searching for any contained opacities in the lumen. The scanning arm can be set to continous motion while multiple sections are taken through the gallbladder at several millimeter intervals. False negative examinations do occur, and this is due to insufficient sections through the gallbladder lumen. At this institution, a 4 percent false negative rate has been found. To minimize this false negative rate, between 100 to 200 sections should be taken through the gallbladder, and although this sounds time-consuming, it must be recalled that each section takes only approximately 2 seconds.

Oblique sections almost perpendicular to the right costal margin are valuable to evaluate the portal vein and the common bile duct. The direction of the portal vein can be noted on the sagittal scans, since there are marked differences in obliquity in different individuals. The portal vein can be seen entering the liver, dividing into left and right branches. In its extrahepatic course, the inferior vena cava is seen posteriorly. The common bile duct (CBD) lies anterior to the portal vein and when traced inferiorly, the CBD dips posteriorly onto the deep surface of the head of the pancreas. At this level, the gastroduodenal artery can also be seen (Fig. 8.2) anterior to the portal vein and passing onto the anterior surface of the pancreas. As the gastroduodenal artery is traced upwards, it becomes continuous with the hepatic artery which ascends with the portal vein and common bile duct to the porta hepatis in the gastrohepatic ligament (p. 98). The pulsation of the hepatic artery (a branch of the celiac trunk) is easily seen by real-time scanning.

Transverse scans can then be obtained again by scanning the gallbladder completely

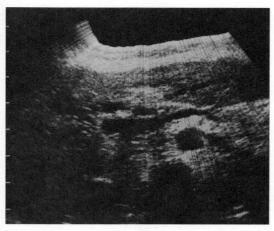
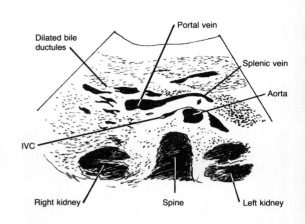

Fig. 8-3. Transverse scan of upper abdomen showing splenic vein passing into the portal vein. This patient has extrahepatic biliary obstruction and dilated bile ducts are seen anterior to the portal vein. Multiple short segments of the biliary tree are seen because of its frequent bifurcation (seen in Fig. 8-1B).

from the neck to the fundus several times. The sonographer should also scan the pancreas with special attention to the head, since the CBD is seen deep to the head of the pancreas. If there is intrahepatic biliary dilatation, the possibility of a carcinoma of the head of the pancreas must be considered, and the level of the obstruction established (pp. 129–136). The size and contour of the CBD are therefore important. Several single sector scans through the anterior margin of the liver over the portal vein should be carried out to evaluate further the state of the intrahepatic ducts (Fig. 8-3).

The portal vein can be seen extending out into the right lobe of the liver. Dilated bile ducts are visualized anterior to it and branching frequently throughout the right and left lobes of the liver. The sonographer should note the position of the gallbladder on transverse scans to confirm its long axis. Once this is established, the scanning arm can be turned obliquely to scan the gallbladder along this axis (Fig. 8-4).

High transverse, intrahepatic gallbladders may be impossible to scan by conventional techniques. This is overcome with a technique of transverse intercostal scanning in the appropriate intercostal space (Fig. 8-5). Intercostal scans in the sagittal plane may also be used (with a 13mm transducer face). The scanning arm is brought far to the patient's

right and angled towards the left so that good skin contact is obtained (Fig. 8-6). The patient is asked to exhale at that time, so that the gallbladder may be raised sufficiently to demonstrate it well. If gas in the duodenum obscures the medial portion of the gallbladder, transverse scans can be carried out with the patient in the right posterior oblique position. In this half-decubitus position any stones in the neck of the gallbladder will descend into the body of the gallbladder away from the air of the duodenum, which may obscure them (Fig. 8-7). Gas in the small bowel and colon can be displaced by deep inspiration, or requesting the patient to blow out the stomach wall.

The upper portion of the common hepatic duct can be visualized lying anterior to the portal vein. This can be seen clearly in the left posterior oblique position, with sagittal scans along the axis of the portal vein (Fig. 8-8).

The size of the common bile duct averages 4 mm with 8 mm being the upper limits of normal in the patient with a gallbladder. After cholecystectomy, the common bile duct is frequently much larger and is said to act as a reservoir. It is still not apparent from the literature whether the common bile duct is dilated before cholecystectomy or subsequent to it.

The left side down decubitus position, can be used to further investigate the nature of

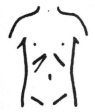

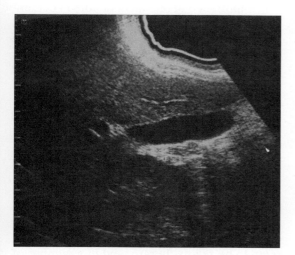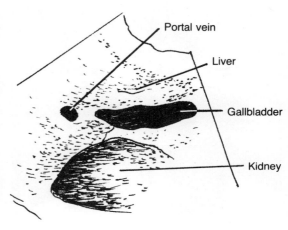

Fig. 8-4. Oblique scan in a plane which is the long axis of the gallbladder. Note that the neck of the gallbladder is always in close proximity to the right branch of the portal vein.

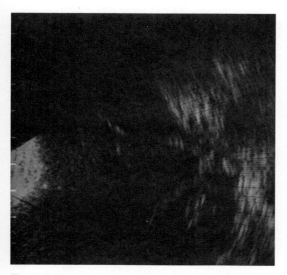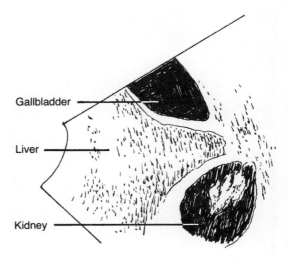

Fig. 8-5. Transverse intercostal scan showing how the liver, right kidney and gallbladder can be visualized. This technique is especially useful in patients with extensive bowel gas or a small liver situated high under the costal margin.

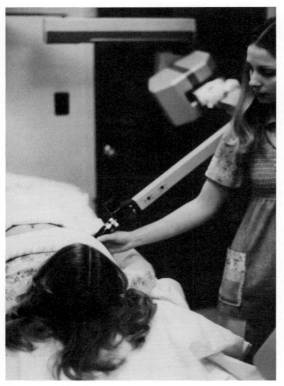

Fig. 8-6. Position of the scanning arm to obtain a near coronal section through the right intercostal spaces. This is a useful scanning technique in patients with copious bowel gas or a small, high liver.

any material demonstrated within the gallbladder lumen. Free movement of an opacity within the gallbladder virtually guarantees that it is a gallstone. The criteria for highly reliable diagnosis of gallstones are as follows: an opacity visualized within the gallbladder lumen; free movement of the opacity with change of position; an acoustic shadow distal to the opacity, due to high attenuation within the gallstone. The importance of technical factors in demonstration of the shadow is discussed later.

Even if no gallstones are apparent, the scans should still be carried out in the decubitus position, so that any small stone imbedded in the neck of the gallbladder may roll into view.

Scans can also be obtained in the erect position in the sagittal plane for the same purpose, although they may be omitted if decubitus scans have demonstrated adequately the pathology, or if the patient is too sick to stand.

If opacities are seen within the gallbladder lumen but do not shadow and cannot be made to shadow, the possibility of nonshadowing stones must be considered. These seem to be relatively rare, and in a number of stones which we have measured, similar attenuation has been found in all. If the opacity

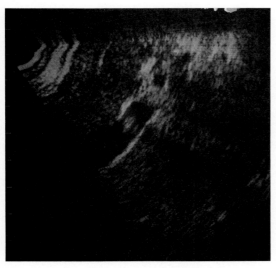

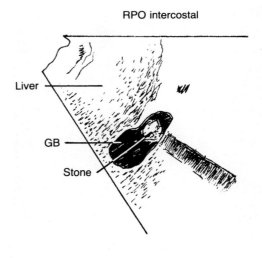

RPO intercostal

Liver

GB

Stone

Fig. 8-7. Intercostal scan with the patient in the right posterior oblique (half decubitus) position. This limited scan nevertheless shows the gallbladder fossa and contained gallstones. Again, this technique may be used successfully to scan patients with small, high livers far under the costal margin.

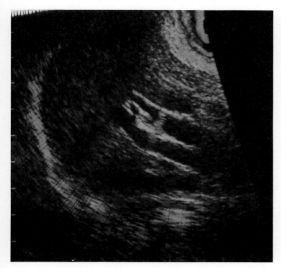 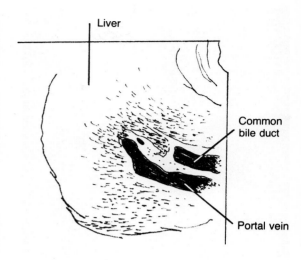

Fig. 8-8. Position suitable for demonstrating the extrahepatic bile ducts and portal vein. Anterior to the portal vein, the common hepatic duct or common bile duct is seen.

does not move with gravity, then a stone may be present but impacted. However, it may also be a polyp or some other fixed pathology of the gallbladder wall, so the same degree of confidence cannot be attached to findings of a non-moving gallstone, as can be associated with a moving stone.

Technical Factors Affecting Acoustical Shadowing

Technical factors may prevent shadowing by at least three different mechanisms, which we have investigated. These include the following technical points:

1. When the gallstone is small compared with the wavelength of the ultrasound beam (0.5 mm at a frequency of 3 MHz), then the ultrasound beam may diffract around it and no shadow is seen distal to the stone.

2. When the gallstone is small compared with the beam width, a shadow may not be apparent distal to it. This problem has been considered in detail to Chapter 3. When a stone is in the focal zone of the transducer, it occludes the beam and produces a shadow. At distances before or beyond the focal zone, shadowing may not be apparent because the gallstone only partially occludes the beam.

3. Distal shadowing may not be apparent if the gain beyond the stone is excessive. This is due to the compression-amplification characteristics of gray-scale systems in which the medium-to-large echoes are greatly compressed in to the very limited dynamic range of a television display (p. 15). Most of the display is given to the low level echoes. Because of this compression of medium and high level echoes, the differences of 12 dB between the stone shadow and the adjacent tissue, may not be apparent on the display if they have been compressed (Figs. 8-9A and B).

Thus, if the stone is small, shadowing will be enhanced by the use of higher frequencies. The stone should lie within the focal zone of the transducer and beam plots should be available to show the narrowest part of the focal zone. Finally, shadowing is enhanced by reduction of the far gain distal to the stone.

Other Gallbladder Contents

Multiple fine stones within the gallbladder may sometimes be seen, which may shadow if they can be collected together in a thick layer by appropriate movement. If they shift rapidly when the patient changes position, they are considered to be gravel. A thick, non-shadowing substance may be seen within the gallblad-

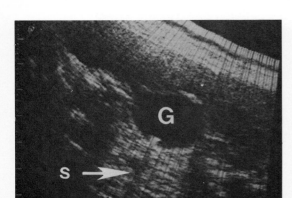

(A)

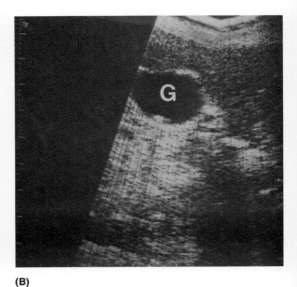

(B)

Fig. 8-9. **(A)** The gallbladder lumen (G) is seen. There is a small opacity within it which shadows distally (S). These appearences are diagnostic of a gallstone. **(B)** Gallbladder lumen (G) is seen. An opacity within the lumen shows no appreciable distal shadow. The distal TGC has been increased and because of the compression amplification, the difference between the shadow and the surrounding tissue has been minimized.

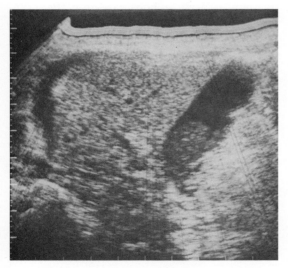

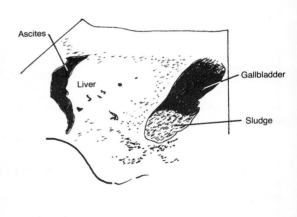

Fig. 8-10. Longitudinal scan of alcoholic patient. Notice that there is ascites between the diaphragm and liver. The gallbladder shows some debris on the dependent surface, which moved slowly, like molasses, with change in patient position.

der, which does not move with gravity, except fairly slowly due to its molasses-like consistency. This is known as sludge (Fig. 8-10). Sludge is fairly common in alcoholics and is of no definite significance.

When the patient has been immobilized for even a few days, it is common to see a small amount of debris within the gallbladder which probably represents inspissated bile. However, it must be stressed that these appearances on ultrasound alone are indistinguishable from those due to pus in the gallbladder, and correlation with clinical history and acute tenderness over the gallbladder area is paramount in making the diagnosis.

Nonvisualization of the Gallbladder on Ultrasound Examination

The most common reason for non-visualization of a dilated gallbladder lumen on ultrasound examination in a fasting patient is that of a diseased gallbladder. Occasionally, the patient has eaten but may deny it, but this will seldom empty the gallbladder completely. When doubt exists, examination should be repeated on the following day. There is a very small incidence of congenital absence of the gallbladder. Thus, for practical purposes, the nonvisualized gallbladder in the truly fasting patient is virtually always diagnostic of disease. The sequence of events is recurrent attacks of acute inflammation of the gallbladder (cholecystitis). The gallbladder wall becomes thickened and more fibrous, and so is incapable of distending during fasting. Usually, these recurrent inflammatory changes are associated with the formation of gallstones. Thus, progression of the disease shows multiple gallstones, often with facets, lying in the gallbladder, which tightly surrounds the contained stones and allows no room for any fluid within the lumen (Fig. 8-11). Occasionally, there may be a small contracted gallbladder without stones. Before concluding definite abnormality of the gallbladder based on ultrasonic nonvisualization, the sonographer should inspect the surface of the abdomen to insure that there is no subcostal incision suggesting the possibility of previous cholecystectomy. The sonographer should also carefully question the patient, and if the patient is mentally confused, question the nurses to ensure that the patient has truly been fasting for at least 8 hours before the examination.

Acute Cholecystitis

This is a diagnostic ultrasound emergency, since some surgeons will proceed to cholecystectomy in these patients. These patients usually complain of severe right upper quadrant pain and tenderness, and the site of maximum tenderness should be established. The sonog-

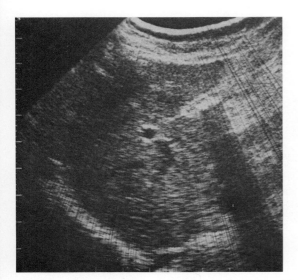
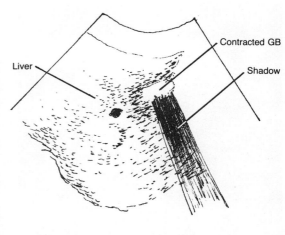

Fig. 8-11. Longitudinal scan through the right lobe of the liver in a fasting patient. There is no evidence of a dilated gallbladder lumen, and the gallbladder fossa is occupied by a highly reflective mass with distal shadowing. In the absence of a normal, physiologically dilated gallbladder lumen, these appearances are highly suspicious of a small, contracted gallbladder full of stones.

rapher should scan over this area and establish whether the site of maximum tenderness coincides with anatomical site of the gallbladder as demonstrated on ultrasound examination. In many of these patients, the gallbladder is noted to have a large number of stones, and in the presence of all this evidence, the diagnosis of acute cholecystitis is very highly probable. However, acalculous cholecystitis can occur,

that is, gallstones are not necessary for the development of acute cholecystitis. The contribution the sonographer then makes is in demonstrating the correlation between the site of maximum tenderness and the site of the gallbladder. Also, the appearance of a subtle echo-free area surrounding the gallbladder lumen has proven to be a valid sign of acute cholecystitis. This may represent edema en-

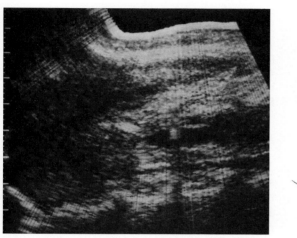
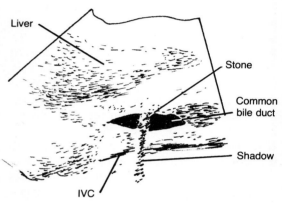

Fig. 8-12. Longitudinal scan through the liver in the plane of the inferior vena cava (IVC). Anterior to the IVC the dilated common bile duct is seen which contains a stone that shadows distally.

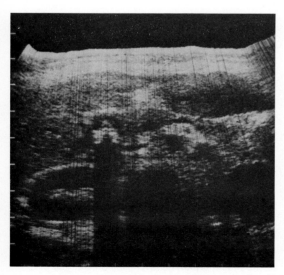
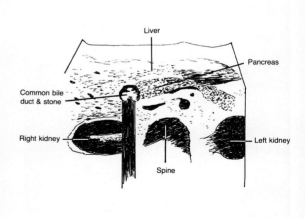

Fig. 8-13. Transverse scan of the upper abdomen. The dilated common bile duct can be seen on the deep surface of the head of the pancreas. Stones are seen within the common bile duct, and these shadow distally. The pancreas, great vessels, left and right kidneys are well seen posteriorly.

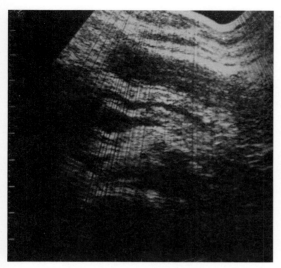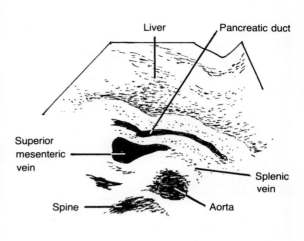

Fig. 8-14. Transverse scan of the pancreas. A dilated pancreatic duct can clearly be seen coursing through the entire gland and running parallel to the splenic vein. This is due to a tumor in the region of the Ampulla of Vater (see Fig. 8-1A).

veloping the gallbladder. In such patients, a recently introduced isotopic scan, employing technetium HIDA seems to be specific. Non-visualization of the gallbladder 30 minutes after injection of this compound is strong evidence of acute cholecystitis. It must be stressed, as with most diagnoses, that the correlation with clinical examination, history and other imaging techniques aids in making the final diagnosis.

Hydrops of the Gallbladder

Hydrops of the gallbladder is a state of acute distention, usually due to obstruction in the neck of the gallbladder or the cystic duct. The gallbladder distends and is usually palpable as a tense mass immediately below the right subcostal margin.

Dilatation of the Intrahepatic Biliary Tree

In the presence of the dilated intrahepatic biliary tree, obstruction (past or present) is implicit and is commonly associated with tumor, stricture, or gallstones. The major importance of ultrasound at present, is the immediate identification of dilated ducts and recognition of this as a surgical cause for jaundice, as op-

posed to intrahepatic conditions such as cirrhosis, multiple metastases or hepatitis.

When dilatation of the intrahepatic biliary tree has been diagnosed, it is important to attempt visualization of the common bile duct using the techniques described, since the level of the obstruction (high near the porta hepatis or low near the pancreas) alters the surgical treatment of these conditions. In at least 50 percent of patients with extrahepatic biliary obstruction, we are able to identify the common bile duct and thereby differentiate high from low obstruction. When the common bile duct can be seen, it can often be traced down to a tumor which may be within the bile duct or pancreas. In these patients, not only the cause of jaundice can be differentiated but also the precise level and type of pathology predicted. In other patients, stones may be seen in the common bile duct (Fig. 8-12). However, one should not always assume that a stone is always the cause of the obstruction, because stones are frequently found in association with obstructing tumors or strictures.

Even with good scanning techniques, common bile duct stones can be missed because ultrasound is a tomographic technique, However, in these patients, intrahepatic biliary dilatation can be seen so that the type of

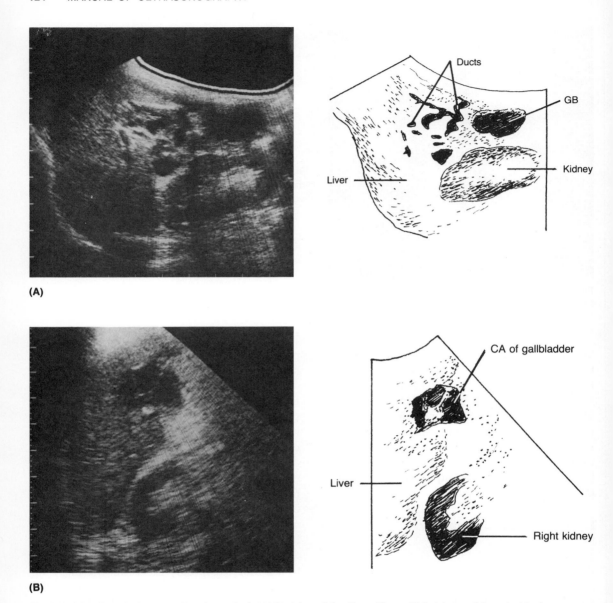

(A)

(B)

Fig. 8-15. **(A)** Parasagittal section through the right lobe of the liver. The gallbladder wall is noted to be markedly thickened and there is definite evidence of dilatation of the entire biliary tree. This proved to be a carcinoma of the gallbladder which had invaded medially and obstructed the common bile duct. **(B)** Limited sector scan in the transverse plane showing the liver, right kidney and abnormal gallbladder. This proved to be a carcinoma of the gallbladder.

jaundice is diagnosed. Scans of the pancreas in the transverse plane may show a dilated common bile duct lying on the deep surface of the head of the pancreas, and the common bile duct may contain a stone which shadows distally (Fig. 8-13). Obstruction in the region of the ampulla of Vater may produce dilatation of the pancreatic duct, in addition to the common bile duct (Fig. 8-14). Carcinoma of the head of the pancreas or other tumors such as lymphomas, carcinoma of the gallbladder or metastases of the lung frequently produce obstruction at the lower end of the common bile duct (Figs. 8-15A and B).

CONCLUSION

The major applications for ultrasound in the biliary tree are the differential diagnosis of jaundice and the diagnosis of gallstones. The noninvasive nature of ultrasound, and the rapidity with which results are obtained economically make ultrasound the logical choice for the initial investigation of the jaundiced patient. In many such patients, the surgical nature of the problem can be recognized and surgery is expedited. In the diagnosis of gallstones, ultrasound competes with oral cholecystography and has similar accuracy. Whereas oral cholecystography may be a suitable screening technique, only in a minority of cases are the gallstones actually displayed. In contast to this, gallstones are virtually always displayed using ultrasound techniques, and this gives a high level of confidence to the imaging technique. Certainly, in those patients

in whom oral cholecystography is contraindicated, ultrasound is the appropriate method.

SUGGESTED READING

Bartrum RJ, Crow HC, Foote SR: Ultrasonic and radiographic cholecystography. NEJM, 538–541, Mr 10, 1977.

Crade M, Taylor KJW, Rosenfield AT, de Graff CS, Minihan P: Surgical and pathologic correlation of cholecystosonography and cholecystography. AJR 131:227-229, 1978.

Jaffe CC, Taylor KJW: Clinical impact of ultrasound beam focussing patterns. Radiology 131:469-472, 1979.

Leevy CM, Popper H, Sherlock S: Diseases of the Liver and Biliary Tract. Standardization of Nomenclature, Diagnostic Criteria and Diagnostic Methodology. DHEW pub. no. 76-725, 1976.

Sherlock S: Diseases of the Liver and Biliary System, 5th Ed. Oxford, Blackwell Scientific, 1975.

Taylor KJW (ed): Diagnostic Ultrasound in Gastrointestinal Disease. New York, Churchill Livingstone, 1979.

Taylor KJW, Jacobson P, Jaffe CC: Lack of an acoustic shadow from gallstones: A possible artifact. Radiology (in press).

White TT, Sarles H, Benhamon J-P: Liver, Bile Ducts and Pancreas. New York, Grune & Stratton, 1977.

9

Pancreas

PAULA JACOBSON

INTRODUCTION

The pancreas is an important retroperitoneal organ which lies obliquely in the upper abdomen, posterior to the liver and stomach, extending from the C-loop of the duodenum to the hilum of the spleen. It is separated from the stomach by the lesser sac of the peritoneum. It is shaped like a tadpole with a bulbous head connected by a neck to the body and tail. The uncinate process of the pancreas is part of the head and lies deep to the superior mesenteric vessels.

Macroscopic Anatomy

The head of the pancreas is enveloped by the C-loop of the duodenum, with the inferior vena cava immediately posterior to it, and the common bile duct grooving the posterior surface of the pancreas before opening into the second (descending) part of the duodenum. The gastroduodenal artery, which is a branch of the hepatic artery, lies on the superficial surface of the head of the pancreas and marks the head of the pancreas as that volume of tissue between the gastroduodenal artery and the common bile duct. The gastroduodenal artery supplies the head of the pancreas by branches from the pancreaticoduodenal loop, which is an arterial arcade following the C-loop of the duodenum.

The uncinate process of the pancreas is a medial projection from the head of the pancreas and lies deep to the superior mesenteric vein (SMV). The SMV separates the uncinate process of the pancreas from the neck. The anatomy of the pancreatic neck, body and tail are best appreciated on transverse scans which show the splenic vein. This vein arches around the prevertebral structures from the hilum of the spleen to join the SMV behind the neck of the pancreas where it forms the portal vein. Thus, the neck of the pancreas is that part of the pancreas anterior to the confluence of the superior mesenteric vein and the splenic vein which forms the portal vein.

The body of the pancreas lies within the stomach bed separated by the cavity of the lesser sac. This is virtually only a slit between the two folds of the peritoneum although it can be seen on an ultrasound scan. The pancreatic body lies anterior to the splenic vein. When the body is traced towards the left, it becomes continuous with the tail of the pancreas which lies in close relation to the hilum of the left kidney and passes in a peritoneal fold towards the hilum of the spleen in the lieno-renal ligament.

Microscopic Anatomy and Physiology

The pancreas is an endocrine as well as exocrine gland. The endocrine part of the pancreas consists of three types of cells which form the Islets of Langerhans. The beta cells are concerned with the production and release of insulin, while the alpha and delta cells produce enzymes called glucagon and gastrin. The exocrine component of the pancreas secretes 1500 to 2000 ml of alkaline juice into the duodenal lumen every 24 hours. This secretion partially neutralizes the acidity of the gastric contents after entry into the duodenum and contains a large number of digestive enzymes that are important in the digestion of proteins, carbohydrates and fats. Many of the protein-splitting enzymes are secreted in inactive form, including trypsinogen and chymostrypsinogin; this prevents digestion of the pancreas by its own enzymes. Amylase is important in carbohydrate breakdown, and the serum amylase levels are useful as an indica-

tor of pancreatitis. The enzyme lipase aids in the digestion of fats but requires bile salts for activation and for detergent action on fat particles to render them water soluble.

Because of the importance of the pancreas in the digestion of both fats and proteins, insufficiency of the exocrine part of the gland is characterized by malabsorption and the formation of fatty stools containing undigested meat fibers. Insufficiency of the endocrine part of the pancreas will lead to insulin deficiency as found in diabetes, particularly of adult onset.

Required Clinical and Laboratory Data

When a patient is referred for pancreatic scanning, the diagnostic sonographer should search for the relevant laboratory values and present these to the interpreting physician with the scan results. Of particular interest in disease of the pancreas are the serum amylase and lipase values. The implications of these enzyme level elevations are summarized in Table 9-1. The normal serum amylase level is less than 70 u/dl. Acute pancreatitis is characterized by a very rapid rise in the serum amylase level to hundreds and even thousands of units; this level declines rapidly towards normal after a few days by inactivation of the enzyme and by urinary excretion. Thus, renal failure may be associated with a raised serum amylase level. A similar cycle is seen in the elevation of serum lipase levels. In alcoholic patients in whom there has been chronic ethanol abuse with subsequent damage to the pancreatic parenchyma, the poorly functioning tissue liberates less amylase and lipase than the normal pancreas. Thus, patients with recurrent pancreatitis and chronic alcoholism have a relatively moderate increase in serum

TABLE 9-1. ENZYME LEVEL ELEVATIONS

	Amylase	Lipase
Normal	<70 u/dl	<1.5 u/ml
Pancreatitis	Rapid rise > 200 u/dl in 8 hours, falling rapidly after 48 hours.	Slow rise > 1.5 u/ml; slower fall than amylase
Pseudocyst	Persistent elevation of amylase and lipase following pancreatitis	

amylase values. The highest levels of serum amylase are seen in non-alcoholic patients who suffer an obstruction of the pancreatic duct. An impacted gallstone, for example, may activate the pancreatic enzymes, though sequestered in the pancreas, and produce a fulminating pancreatitis of great severity. These patients are gravely ill and may be in shock. Serum amylase levels may exceed 5000 u/dl, and a substantial mortality occurs. Such patients are also prime candidates for the development of a subsequent pancreatic pseudocyst. Other causes of pseudocysts are past surgery and trauma. A patient having cystic fibrosis may also have one or more cysts within the pancreas.

The clinical state of the patient should be observed, noting any evidence of emaciation which is common in chronic alcoholics and is virtually universal in cases of advanced pancreatic malignancy. The referring physician should inform the sonographer about such symptoms as nausea, vomiting, weight loss and back pain, which are frequent though non-specific accompaniments of pancreatic disease. If the clinical state is not provided, it should be solicited and noted by the sonographer.

SCANNING TECHNIQUES

Scans of the pancreas are commenced by adjusting the gain setting to write normal pancreatic parenchyma. Gain settings are lower than those used for the liver since the pancreas is more highly echogenic. After liberally coating the upper abdomen with mineral oil, scanning is begun in the sagittal plane. A smooth, single-sector scan is performed, using the left lobe of the liver as an acoustic window to the pancreas. If air is encountered before the level of the pancreas, the patient is asked to inspire deeply, thus depressing the diaphragm and bringing the liver down over the pancreatic area. The body of the pancreas is seen on sagittal sections anterior to the aorta between the celiac trunk and the superior mesenteric artery (SMA) (Fig. 9-1). Further parasagittal sections towards the left demonstrate the tail of the pancreas at the level of the splenic vein and the left renal vein (Fig. 9-2). Usually the entire tail is not demonstrated on these views. Further parasagittal scans to the right of the midline show the neck of the pancreas lying superficial to the superior mesenteric vein (SMV) and the uncinate process of the pancreas lying deep to it (Fig. 9-3). Slightly further towards the right, a paramedian section shows the inferior vena cava (IVC); anterior to the IVC is the head of the pancreas.

Transverse scans should be carried out in the light of the findings on the parasagittal scans. If gas was noted throughout the stomach and bowel, the scanning arm can be angled caudally 10 to 15 degrees, thereby using the liver as an acoustic window to visualize the pancreas in a lower plane. If gas is seen in the stomach, but not inferiorly, the scanning arm may be angled cephalad to gain access to the pancreas. The scanning arm should be arranged transversely or obliquely, with the right side of the sections lower than the left and therefore approximately parallel to the longitudinal axis of the pancreas.

It must be stressed, as with all ultrasound scanning, that rigid adherence to scanning techniques based on precise anatomical landmarks is impractical. The sonographer must find areas that are free of gas and scan through them to the organ of interest. Nuclear medicine studies of the pancreas have indicated that there are vast variations in the overall contour of the pancreas, which again will prohibit rigid, stereotyped scanning techniques.

Transverse scanning is commenced immediately below the xiphisternum, and the various anatomical structures recognized in progressively caudal sequential scans, until the important vascular landmarks are identified. A transverse section carried out immediately below the xiphisternum shows the celiac trunk and its branches (Fig. 9-4). Inferior to this plane, the splenic vein is recognized arching around the prevertebral structures to join the mesenteric vein, forming the portal vein. This confluence of veins lies posterior to the neck of the pancreas, so that the echogenic area immediately anterior to the splenic vein is the neck, body and tail of the pancreas (Fig. 9-

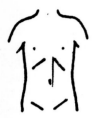

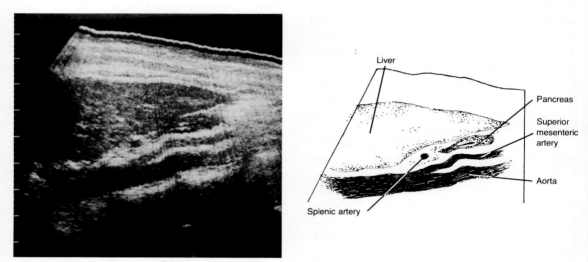

Fig. 9-1. Longitudinal section in the plane of the aorta showing the origin of the superior mesenteric artery. The splenic artery is seen passing towards the left. The pancreas is seen anterior to the superior mesenteric artery.

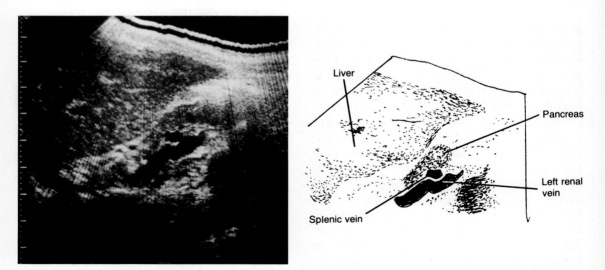

Fig. 9-2. Longitudinal section to the left of the aorta. The splenic vein and left renal vein are seen, with the pancreas situated superficially, and posterior to the left lobe of the liver.

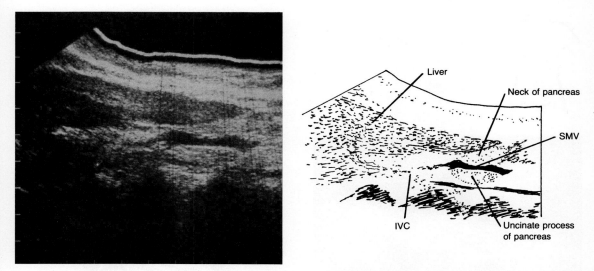

Fig. 9-3. Longitudinal section in the plane of the inferior vena cava (IVC). The superior mesenteric vein (SMV) is well seen. Superficial to the SMV is the densely reflective neck of the pancreas, while deep to it is the uncinate process.

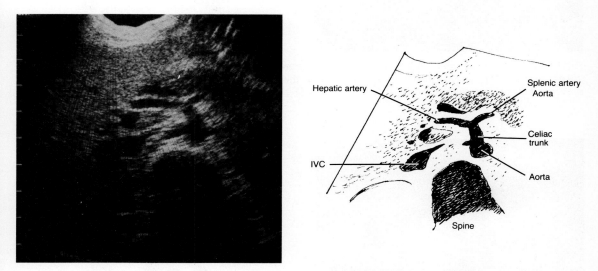

Fig. 9-4. Transverse scan showing the celiac trunk emerging from the aorta and dividing into the hepatic artery passing towards the right, and the splenic artery passing towards the left. The inferior vena cava is seen receiving the left renal vein. The portal vein is seen between the inferior vena cava and the hepatic artery.

5). The scanning arm can now be adjusted to a more oblique position so that the pancreas and splenic vein are seen in their entirety. The head of the pancreas is then seen lying slightly inferior to the junction of the splenic vein and SMV at the level of the left renal vein. The head of the pancreas has a highly constant re-lationship to the duodenal loop and lies within its concavity. In ultrasound scans, the duode-num is seen either as a fluid-filled structure frequently containing some echogenic debris, or as an air-filled structure which shadows dis-tally (Fig. 9-6A and B). Lateral to the duode-num, the distended gallbladder is seen, while

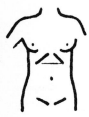

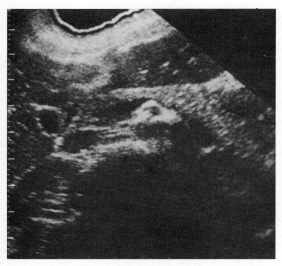

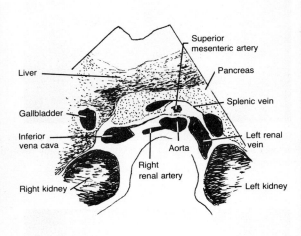

Fig. 9-5. Transverse scan through the upper abdomen showing the splenic vein forming the portal vein by joining the superior mesenteric vein behind the neck of the pancreas. The head of the pancreas is seen as a bulbous mass projecting towards the right.

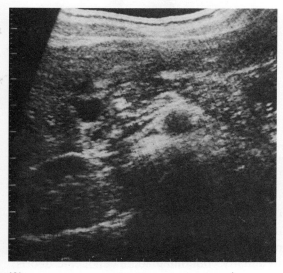

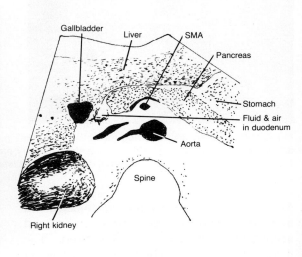

(A)

Fig. 9-6. **(A)** Transverse scan of the upper abdomen with fluid in the fundus of the stomach and duodenum. The head, neck, body and tail of the pancreas are well displayed and the great vessels are seen posteriorly.

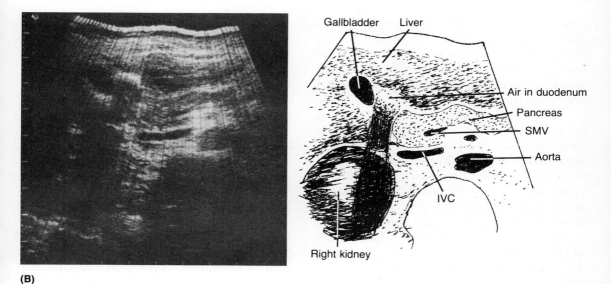

(B)

Fig. 9-6. (continued) **(B)** Transverse scan showing the pancreas and great vessels. Air in the duodenum is seen between the gallbladder laterally and head of the pancreas medially.

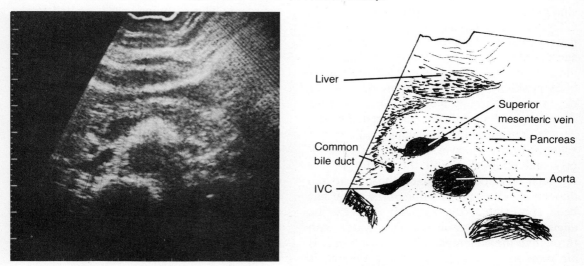

Fig. 9-7. Transverse scan of the upper abdomen to show the pancreas with the common bile duct (CBD) on the deep surface of the head of the pancreas.

medial to the duodenum, the typical echogenic parenchyma of the pancreatic head is seen. In this position, the common bile duct is recognized as a small sonolucent structure just lateral to the SMV—and lying on the deep surface of the head of the pancreas (Fig. 9-7). To visualize the head of the pancreas better when it is obscured by gas, a 45 degree right posterior oblique scan done transversely may shift the duodenum to the right enough to reveal the head and body of the pancreas in their entirety.

The tail of the pancreas is poorly visualized from the anterior aspect, and often it is necessary to place the patient prone and to scan the tail of the pancreas using the left kidney as an acoustic window. The echogenic tail of the pancreas is seen lying on the superficial surface of the kidney. There are, however, wide variations in this anatomical relationship, and although the pancreas is described anatomically as being in apposition to the hilum of the kidney, the tail is frequently seen at a higher or lower level.

If the routine scans of the pancreas using the above technique are unsuccessful due to excessive abdominal gas, the sonographer can use a method recently described from this center, involving water distention of the stomach. When the fundus of the stomach is distended with a large quantity of water, the tail of the pancreas will appear sandwiched between it and the left kidney. It should be noted that the stomach is in an immediate anterior relation to the pancreas, that is, the pancreas lies in the stomach bed. Thus, air contained within the body and antrum of the stomach may obscure visualization of the pancreas. This relationship of the stomach to the pancreas is used in CT scanning by having the patient drink contrast medium which outlines the superficial surface of the pancreas. For ultrasound scanning, the patient lies on the left side (left decubitus position), and drinks approximately 12 oz. of water through a straw, which reduces the number of air bubbles generated. The patient is then turned to the supine position and scanned in the transverse plane, both superiorly and inferiorly, until the fundus of the stomach has been visualized through to the duodenum. Once the position of the water has been appreciated, the scanning arm can be angled to use the stomach as a water path through to the pancreas in the stomach bed. If air remains in the stomach, the patient is turned to the right posterior oblique position, and air bubbles may then rise to the fundus and permit visualization of the head, body and sometimes tail of the pancreas. Once the air bubbles disperse, slightly left posterior oblique, transverse scans with a slightly cephalad angulation of the arm, can be obtained to delineate the entire tail. The dramatic improvement that may be obtained by this technique is shown in Fig. 9-8A and B.

If the pancreatic area is still obscured by air in the stomach, the patient is scanned in the erect position. The patient stands facing the stretcher, and the arm of the ultrasound equipment is rotated so that it is almost horizontal. In this position, transverse scans can be carried out. It may be necessary to reverse the orientation of the image, so that the right side of the patient still appears on the left side of the screen. In this position, the relationship of the stomach relative to the pancreas must again be determined, and the position of the scanning arm must be adjusted accordingly. Any air bubbles in the stomach will tend to rise to the fundus allowing the entire pancreas to be seen (Fig. 9-9).

One further technique is used at this institution to visualize the tail of the pancreas. When water can be seen in the fundus and body of the stomach on supine scans, the tail of the pancreas can be scanned along the plane of its long axis. This is accomplished by noting the angle the tail makes on the transverse water scans. The scanning arm is angled to the same degree before turning into the sagittal plane and scanning past the SMA and aorta. The tail of the pancreas is seen as in Figure 9-10, with water superficial to it in the fundus of the stomach and the body of the stomach below it. For this scanning technique, the water must be essentially free of air bubbles. This projection is most useful in proving the presence of a mass in the tail of the pancreas and differentiating it from masses in the gut, bowel or mesentery.

When a patient is referred for a pancreatic examination, it is important to scan the rest of the upper abdomen. Other diseases may coexist with disease of the pancreas, and although the pancreas may not be the cause of the symptoms and signs, pathology may be demonstrated in adjacent organs (see chaps. on liver, gallbladder, and biliary tree). Since alcoholic changes in the liver, such as alcoholic hepatitis, fatty infiltration and cirrhosis, are frequently found in association with pancreatitis and carcinoma of the pancreas, the liver also must be carefully scanned.

The gallbladder and biliary tree must also be visualized in a pancreatic examination. The presence of gallstones may be incidental, but they may produce acute pancreatitis by passing down the common bile duct and becoming

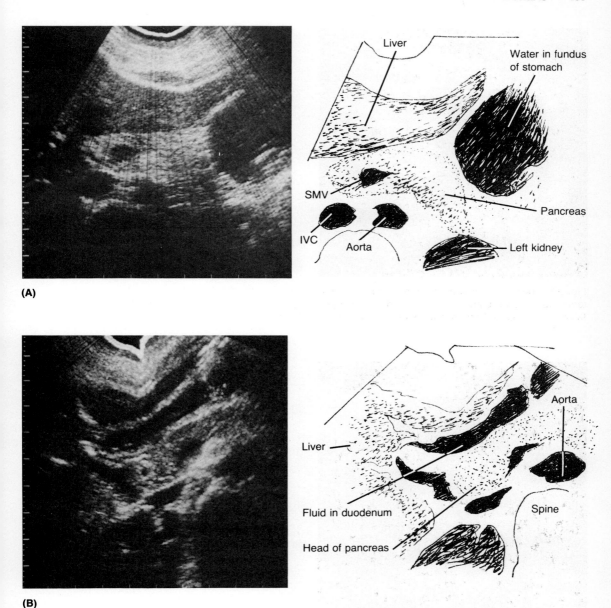

Fig. 9-8. **(A)** Transverse section through the upper abdomen to show the pancreas with water in the fundus of the stomach. Notice that the pancreas lies in the stomach bed and therefore can be well outlined by adequate water in the stomach. **(B)** Sections through the upper abdomen showing the entire pancreas with the exception of the tail. The pancreas is well outlined by water in the gastric fundus, antrum and duodenum.

impacted in the Ampulla of Vater, the common entrance for both the biliary tree and the pancreatic duct into the duodenum. If a gallstone is impacted in this position, bile enters the pancreas and activates the digestive enzymes. A disease follows which varies in severity from moderate epigastric pain, to shock, hemorrhage, necrosis and death. In non-alcoholics when the cause of pancreatitis is not immediately apparent, gallstones should

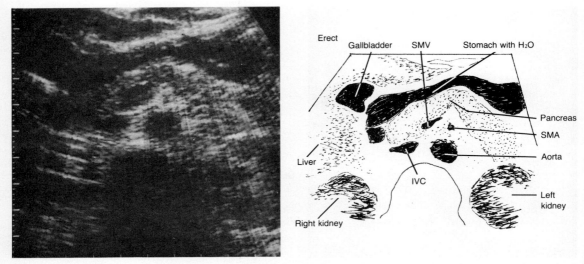

Fig. 9-9. Transverse scan of the upper abdomen with the patient upright. This is a particularly valuable technique to scan patients with obscuring bowel gas, despite the use of the water technique. The stomach is filled with water and outlines the stomach bed in which the pancreas lies.

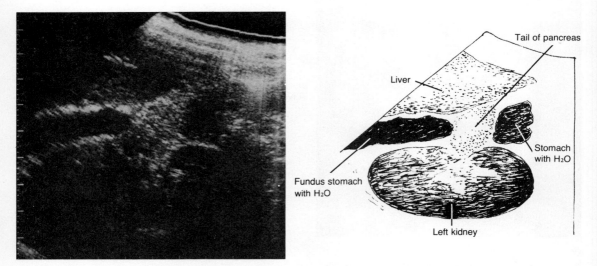

Fig. 9-10. Oblique scan in the plane of the tail of the pancreas. The left kidney is seen posteriorly. Water is seen in the fundus of the stomach, and the tail of the pancreas is seen in contact with the hilum of the left kidney.

be considered early in the differential diagnosis and excluded by ultrasound scanning (Fig. 9-11 and 9-12).

Carcinoma of the head of the pancreas also causes obstruction to the common bile duct, which is embedded on the posterior aspect of the pancreas. The patient with carci-noma of the head of the pancreas typically has a history of weight loss and jaundice. The demonstration of a dilated biliary tree and a mass in the head of the pancreas suggests a carcinoma of the head of the pancreas (a carcinoma of the body of the pancreas is shown in Fig. 9-13).

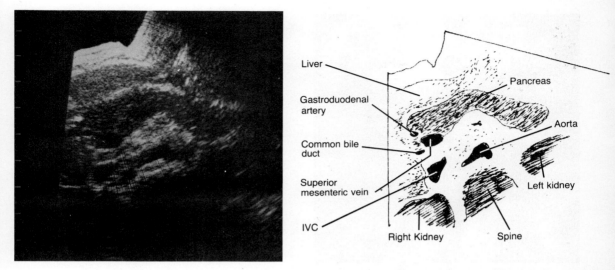

Fig. 9-11. Transverse sector scan through the pancreas in a patient with pancreatitis. Note that the pancreas is less echogenic than the liver, which is situated superficial to the pancreas. Lateral to the formation of the portal vein, the common bile duct is seen on the deep surface of the head of the pancreas, and the gastroduodenal artery is seen on the superficial surface.

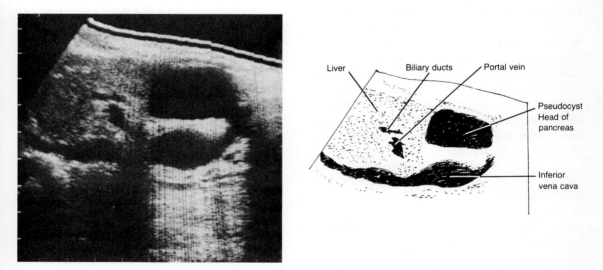

Fig. 9-12. Longitudinal scan in the plane of the inferior vena cava showing a large prevertebral cystic mass, consistent with a pseudocyst in the head of the pancreas.

Rarer types of tumors do occur and may be diagnosed by ultrasound. One such tumor, an islet cell tumor, which may be either a benign or malignant growth, arises from the islet cells of the pancreas. It may produce excessive gastrin, an enzyme that stimulates the acid-producing parietal cells of the stomach.

Patients suffering from this disease (Zollinger-Ellison syndrome), present with intractable ulceration of the stomach, duodenum and jejunum. CT scanning in these patients is probably more sensitive; surgery is curative. Other islet cell tumors may occur which do not secrete excessive gastrin—but are charac-

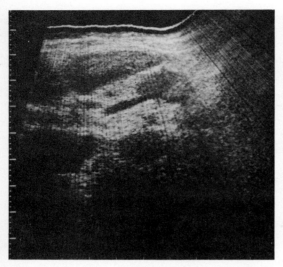 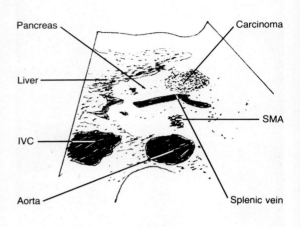

Fig. 9-13. Transverse scan through the pancreas. Notice that there is some enlargement and a definite abnormality of consistency in the body of the pancreas. This suggests either localized pancreatitis or more likely, a carcinoma of the pancreas.

terized by severe and unrelenting diarrhea.

An insulin-secreting adenoma may cause bizarre symptoms, such as loss of consciousness or psychotic behavior, due to oversecretion of insulin. Insulin excess produces hypoglycemia and results in recurrent loss of consciousness. Nonfunctioning, benign tumors, such as adenomas may also occur, producing few symptoms until their size causes pressure on surrounding organs.

CONCLUSION

It must be stressed that flexibility in scanning techniques is a major requirement for successfully scanning the pancreas. The placement of the sections must be determined in light of the information obtained from earlier sections. Gas pockets must be identified and avoided, and acoustic windows must be actively sought by an intelligent scanning approach. With a

flexible and imaginative scanning technique, the pancreas can be visualized in 90 percent of the population. In emaciated patients lacking retroperitoneal fat, with chronic inflammatory or malignant pancreatic disease, ultrasound visualization may be superior to that obtained by computerized tomography. Thus, the clinician must rely heavily on the excellence achieved by the sonographer.

SUGGESTED READING

Crade M, Taylor KJW, Rosenfield AT: Water distention of the gut in the evaluation of the pancreas by ultrasound. AJR 131:348-349, 1978.

de Graaff CS, Taylor KJW, Simonds BD, Rosenfield AT: Grey scale echography of the pancreas: re-evaluation of normal size. Radiology 129:167-171, 1978.

Taylor KJW (ed): Diagnostic Ultrasound in Gastrointestinal Disease. New York, Churchill Livingstone, 1979.

White TT, Sarles H, Behnamon J-P: Liver, Bile Ducts and Pancreas. New York, Grune & Stratton, 1977.

10

Renal Ultrasonography

CAROL A. TALMONT

INTRODUCTION

Gray-scale ultrasound provides a non-invasive and immediate way to study the kidneys and perirenal region. Ultrasound should be used as a complementary study along with other diagnostic modalities and the clinical history to achieve an accurate diagnosis. Other accompanying diagnostic examinations include intravenous pyelography (IVP) with nephrotomography, retrograde pyelography, isotope studies especially for renal function, and most recently computerized axial tomography (CT). In patients with a history of allergic reaction to iodine based contrast media, ultrasound should be used as the initial examination. In most other patients, ultrasound is performed as a complementary study to the urogram (IVP), either to investigate further the nature of a mass visualized, or to clarify an equivocal result.

Using ultrasound, renal size can be determined and fluid or solid renal masses can be differentiated. During scanning of the right kidney, the surrounding organs are also imaged and incidental pathology of the gallbladder and liver can be noted. The ureters, unless grossly dilated, are not usually visualized with ultrasound instrumentation currently available.

Clinical Data

The clinical history provides an indication for further studies or assistance in making the final diagnosis. Relatively early symptoms and signs of renal disease may include: hematuria, polyuria, oliguria, generalized edema, urgency, pain and palpable renal masses. There may be acute onset of renal failure. On the basis of these signs and symptoms, and the results of ultrasound examination and other diagnostic procedures, differential diagnosis will be narrowed. Frequently, there are no such obvious symptoms and signs, and the first evidence of disease is the insidious onset of renal failure.

The important serum levels for the diagnosis of renal failure are the blood urinary nitrogen (BUN), and creatinine. The normal BUN is 10-15 mg percent and serum creatinine is less than 1.5 mg percent. The kidneys show immense reserve, and loss of up to 60 percent of functioning renal parenchyma will lead to no elevation of either BUN or creatinine. Increased protein in urine is another indicator of disease. Thus, when these levels are elevated renal function is severely impaired.

Anatomy

The kidneys are located in the retroperitoneal region of the abdominal cavity, one on either side of the spine. The kidneys are surrounded by adipose tissue (perirenal fat) and dense connective tissue (Gerota's fascia). The perirenal fat produces a characteristic bright echogenic appearance on ultrasound imaging. The kidneys rest on the psoas major and quadratus lumborum muscles and on part of the diaphragm. Although they are supported by renal fascia, they are not rigidly fixed and move with the diaphragm during respiration. This renal movement, as well as the pulsations of the large renal arteries and veins can be appreciated on real-time ultrasound scanning.

The kidney is bean-shaped; its lateral border is convex and the medial border concave. In the central portion of the concave border, there is a deep longitudinal fissure known as the *hilus* where the vessels and nerves enter and leave, and from where the ureter extends downward towards the urinary bladder.

Three major sections of the kidney should be seen on ultrasound scanning: cortex, pelvis and medulla (Fig. 10-1). The renal cortex, or outer portion of the kidney, arches over the pyramids of the medulla and dips between adjacent pyramids. These inward extensions of the cortical substance are called the *renal columns* (of Bertin).

The renal pelvis is a funnel shaped sac that forms the upper expanded end of the ureter. It receives urine from all parts of the kidney via the calyces, which are cup-shaped extensions of the renal pelvis. Renal calculi may form in the pelvis of the kidney and may cause pain and hematuria.

The renal medulla consists of striated, cone-shaped structures called the *renal pyramids*. These vary in number, but there are usually twelve in each kidney. The base of each pyramid is directed toward the cortex, and the apex projects as a papilla into the calyces of the renal pelvis.

Blood is conveyed to each kidney through the renal artery which gives off the lobar arteries, usually one to each pyramid. Each lobar branch gives off two to three interlobar arteries which pass between adjacent pyramids and give off small branches to the glomeruli as they extend toward the cortex. The glomeruli are the sites of blood filtration. The interlobar arteries give off the arcuate arteries which cross at the junction of the cortex and medulla. After passing through the glomeruli, blood flows through the efferent arterioles into the capillary beds that surround the renal tubules; these microscopic networks are called the peritubular capillaries. When leaving the peritubular capillaries, blood flows into stellate veins and then into the interlobular veins. The veins that drain the kidneys follow the same general course as the arteries that lie beside them. (Fig. 10-2).

ULTRASONIC APPEARANCES OF RENAL PARENCHYMA AND THE RENAL SINUS

The arcuate vessels within the renal parenchyma are generally seen in the transverse plane or oblique section at the corticomedullary junction (Figs. 10-3 and 4). They can be visualized in approximately 50 percent of patients. The normal cortex contains echoes while the medulla is more sonolucent (Fig. 10-5). The normal cortex and medulla can be clearly differentiated in most patients. A high frequency transducer should be employed to delineate

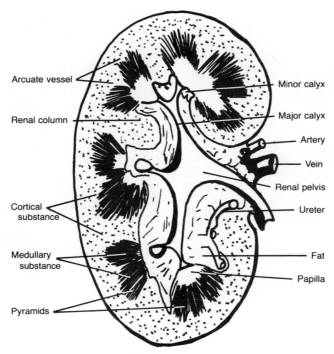

Fig. 10-1. Longitudinal section through the kidney showing the detailed macroscopical anatomy.

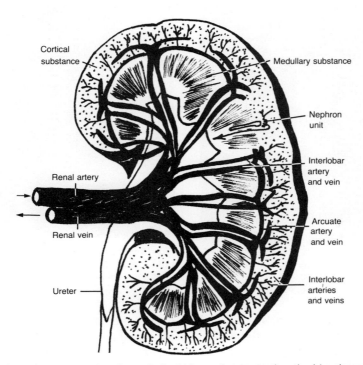

Fig. 10-2. Schema of longitudinal section through the kidney, demonstrating the blood supply and venous drainage of the kidney.

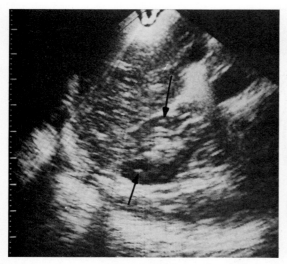

Fig. 10-3. Transverse section through the right upper quadrant showing the right kidney lying posterior to the liver. The arcuate vessels are arrowed, and lie at the junction of the cortex and medulla.

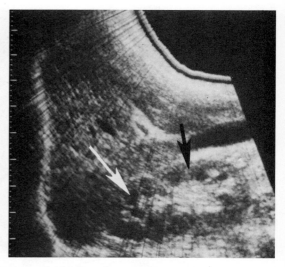

Fig. 10-5. Section through the longitudinal axis of the right kidney. The pyramids (white arrow) are less echogenic than the surrounding cortex (black arrow). Notice that the gallbladder is most frequently anterior to the lower pole of the right kidney, and the liver lies anterior to the upper pole of the right kidney.

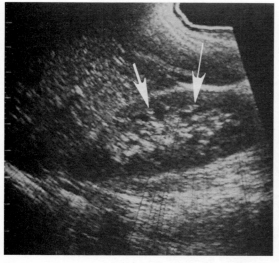

Fig. 10-4. Scan through the longitudinal axis of the right kidney. Notice the pyramids are less echogenic than the cortex of the kidney. The arcuate vessels are arrowed.

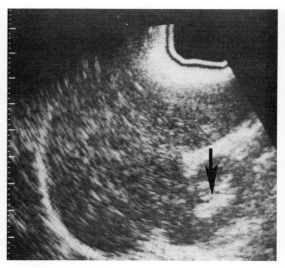

Fig. 10-6. Longitudinal section through the liver and right kidney. Note that the renal sinus contains very high level echoes (arrowed).

sharp corticomedullary definition. The normal cortex appears less echogenic than the parenchyma of the liver, except in the presence of liver disease. The renal sinus returns high level echoes on gray-scale echography (Fig. 10-

6), and the infundibula and calyces can also be identified and evaluated. Normal calyces vary in size, and the appearances of the collecting system vary with the degree of hydration (Fig. 10-7). Renal stones may be identified within

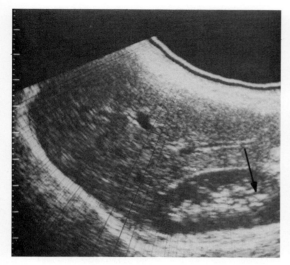

Fig. 10-7. Longitudinal scan through the liver and right kidney. A fine extension from the renal pelvis is seen which is called the infundibula (arrowed); this ends in a cup into which the renal papilla projects. These prolongations from the renal sinus constitute the lesser calyces.

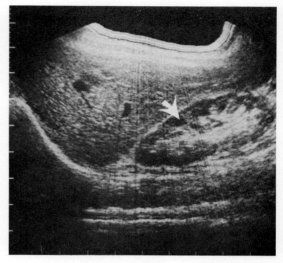

Fig. 10-8. Longitudinal section through the liver and right kidney by a simple-sector scan. The liver is separated from the kidney by the perirenal fat and Gerota's fascia. The pyramids (arrowed) can be delineated. Centrally is the echogenic renal sinus.

the renal sinus, particularly if acoustic shadowing is seen.

SCANNING TECHNIQUES

To scan the kidneys, a coupling agent of mineral oil, or in patients with surgical wounds, acoustical gel, is used. A transducer with the highest frequency that will penetrate the patient should be employed, but one may need to change frequencies to obtain resolution in different projections. A narrow faced transducer is best suited for obtaining intercostal scans. Appropriate gain settings and TGC display are important factors to consider in the evaluation of the renal parenchyma. The gain setting should be such that the liver parenchyma is displayed with even consistency. The renal cortex should be well visualized and the medulla appreciated as a sonolucent structure.

The patient should first be placed in the supine position for scanning the right kidney. The liver is used as an acoustic window to aid in the visualization of the renal parenchyma. Longitudinal, parasagittal sector scans are obtained by arching the transducer, beginning under the ribs in a single linear or sector scan, to the inferior portion of the kidney. The patient should suspend respiration to displace the liver and kidney inferiorly and to avoid artifacts (Fig. 10-8).

The sonographer should scan the right kidney from its most medial portion to its most lateral portion, using the continuous survey mode — not specific one or two centimeter sections. Scans demonstrating pathology should be recorded along with scans identifying normal renal parenchyma. The right kidney should then be examined in the transverse plane. Simply maneuver the arm of the system to the left side of the patient; the patient remains in the supine position. The transducer is placed intercostally and a single-sector arc is produced. The sonographer should begin at the most superior portion of the kidney and scan continuously inferior using the survey mode. Scans at several levels should be obtained, and scans should be recorded at the upper pole, renal pelvis and lower pole (Fig. 10-9). The sonographer may need to scan between various intercostal spaces to delineate different sections of the kidney, or request

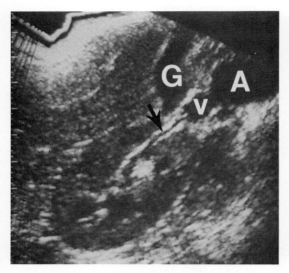

Fig. 10-9. Transverse sector scan through the liver, right kidney and gallbladder (G). The right renal vein (arrowed) can be seen draining into the inferior vena cava (V). More medially the aorta (A) is seen.

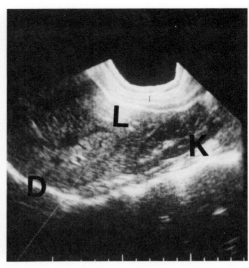

Fig. 10-10. Coronal scan obtained with the patient in the left decubitus position. The right kidney (K) is seen below the liver (L) and diaphragm (D).

the patient to suspend respiration at different degrees of inhalation.

The right kidney is then approached with the patient in the left decubitus position (right side up). The transducer is placed intercostally along the midaxillary line in the coronal plane. A single-sector arc is made encompassing the right hemidiaphragm, the liver and right kidney (Fig. 10-10). Scans are obtained along this coronal axis from the posterior aspect of the patient to the anterior aspect, on the survey mode. This decubitus projection may be helpful in identifying lesions not recognized in other projections.

The left kidney is best demonstrated with the patient in the right decubitus position (left side up). This avoids overlying gas which would be visualized with the patient in the supine position. Coronal sector scans as previously described are obtained at several levels from the posterior aspect of the patient to the anterior aspect (Fig. 10-11).

Routine scans with the patient prone should be included. Transverse sector scans lateral to the spine are obtained. Beginning at the superior portion of the kidneys, the sonographer may mark the patient's skin

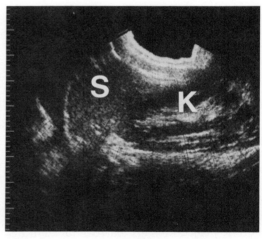

Fig. 10-11. Coronal scan of the left kidney with the patient in the right decubitus position. The spleen (S) is used as an acoustic window to the left subphrenic space and upper pole of the left kidney (K).

with a wax pencil where the collecting system is seen. This will appear as an echogenic area in the medial portion of the kidney. Scans are obtained at the level of the upper pole, mid-portion, and lower pole (Fig. 10-12). From these skin marks, the exact longitudinal lie of the kidney is identified.

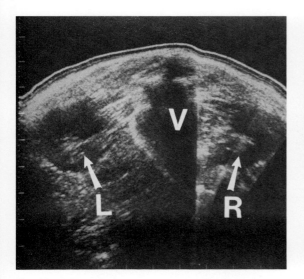

Fig. 10-12. Transverse sector scan with the patient in the prone position. The left (L) and right (R) kidneys can be seen using this technique. The vertebra (V) is seen between the kidneys. Note that there is very poor renal detail using this technique. Considerable scattering of the beam occurs in the subcutaneous fatty tissues, but in addition, the kidneys are not in the focal zone of the transducer.

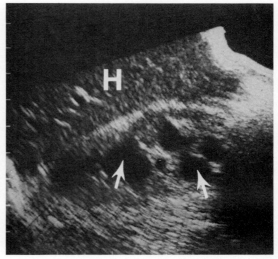

Fig. 10-13. Longitudinal scan through the right kidney and right lobe of the liver (H). Multiple lobulated, fluid-filled spaces are seen filling the renal pelvis. These appearances are characteristic of mild hydronephrotic changes.

Pathology

A perinephric abscess can be readily identified on ultrasound as a sonolucent area surrounding the kidney. Once this collection is identified, the fluid may be aspirated (p. 173).

Hydronephrosis can be easily diagnosed by ultrasound, and appears as dilatation of the collecting system. The normal intrarenal central echoes become separated, and as dilatation becomes more marked, a sonolucent area is seen (Fig. 10-13). The dilated pelvicalyceal system appears as a lobulated echo free area in cases of severe hydronephrosis. Minimal hydronephrosis is commonly seen in the pregnant patient.

Ultrasound is extremely useful in the investigation of renal masses, and is particularly helpful in differentiating solid masses from renal cysts. Solid tumors have internal echoes when high gain is employed, with a decrease in posterior wall echoes due to tissue attenuation (Fig. 10-14). Malignant tumors usually demonstrate irregular walls. Renal cysts are char-acteristically sonolucent with a flat A-scan. The echoes of the posterior wall are enhanced and the walls are smooth (Fig. 10-15). Renal cyst punctures are performed under ultrasound guidance, as discussed in pp. 179–182.

Polycystic kidney disease is a hereditary disorder characterized by multiple cysts in both kidneys which destroy the surrounding parenchyma. Ultrasound is an excellent modality for the visualization of renal cysts (Fig. 10-16). In one-third of patients with polycystic kidney disease there is accompanying cystic involvement of other organs, primarily the liver.

Ultrasound is also used as a means for following up patients with transplanted kidneys, as there is little discomfort and no exposure to ionizing radiation. Renal transplants are usually placed along the ileopsoas margins in the iliac fossa, and can be examined by ultrasound for signs of obstruction or rejection. Clinical signs of rejection are fever, low urine output, hypertension, pain and tenderness over the surgical site. On ultrasound examination there will be a change in echogenicity of the parenchyma and a change in renal size. The cortex of the rejecting kidney gener-

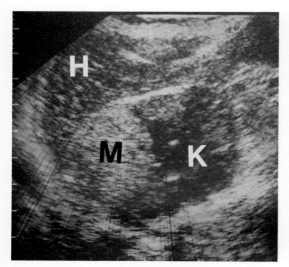

Fig. 10-14. Longitudinal scan through the right kidney (K). Note that the upper pole has an extensive echogenic irregular mass, consistent with a tumor. Such appearances are frequently found in carcinoma of the kidney. There was no evidence of surrounding liver involvement (H). In such patients, the inferior vena cava and renal vein should be carefully searched for any sign of tumor extension.

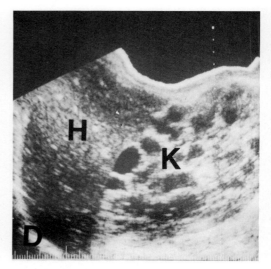

Fig. 10-16. Longitudinal scan of the liver (H) and right kidney (K). Note the extensive replacement of the kidney by multiple cysts in a patient with polycystic kidney disease. The right hemidiaphragm is seen above (D).

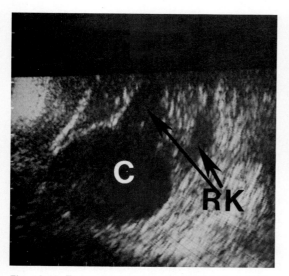

Fig. 10-15. Transverse scan of the right kidney (RK). A large echo-free mass (C) is seen extending out from the kidney.

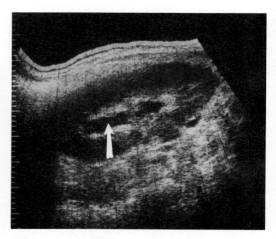

Fig. 10-17. Longitudinal scan of an obstructed, transplanted kidney showing dilatation of the renal sinus (arrowed).

ally shows increased echo amplitude. In the patient with an obstructed transplant, the renal pelvis shows marked dilatation of the renal sinus (Fig. 10-17). Ultrasound is also used to diagnose lymphoceles and urinomas which may occur after transplant.

End stage kidneys are often evaluated in ultrasound studies. Among the many causes for this condition are infection due to pyelonephritis, chronic reflux, immunologic disorders, glomerulonephritis, diabetes, and vascular diseases such as atherosclerosis. Ultrasound

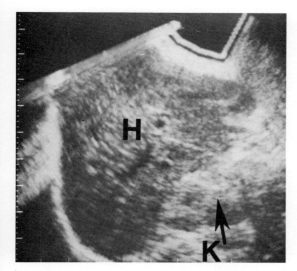

Fig. 10-18. Longitudinal scan through the liver (H) and right kidney (K). Notice that the kidney is highly echogenic and is small in overall size. These appearances are consistent with end stage medical renal disease.

demonstrates small kidneys and echogenic parenchyma due to the presence of fibrous tissue (Fig. 10-18).

SUGGESTED READING

Clinics In Diagnostic Ultrasound, Vol. 2, (ed.) A.T. Rosenfield. Churchill Livingstone, New York, 1979.

Cook JH III, Rosenfield AT, Taylor KJW: Ultrasonic demonstration of intrarenal anatomy. AJR 129:831-835, 1977.

Kay CJ, Rosenfield AT, Taylor KJW, et al: Ultrasonic characteristics of chronic atrophic pyelonephritis. AJR 132:47-49, 1979.

Rosenfield AT, Taylor KJW: Gray-scale nephrosonography: current status. J Urol 117:2-6, 1977.

Rosenfield AT, Taylor KJW, Crade M, et al: Anatomy and pathology of the kidney by gray-scale ultrasound. Radiology 128:737-744, 1978.

Sagel SS, Stanley RJ, Levitt RG, et al: Computed tomography of the kidney. Radiology 124:359-370, 1977.

Stables DP, Ginsberg NJ, Johnson ML: Percutaneous nephrostomy: a series and review of the literature. AJR 130:75−82, 1978.

11

Abscesses

CAROL A. TALMONT

INTRODUCTION

The diagnosis and localization of abdominal and pelvic abscesses presents a serious problem in clinical practice. Due to delay in diagnosis, a mortality rate of 30 percent may result, despite adequate drainage and antibiotic therapy. Gray-scale ultrasound instrumentation has contributed greatly to the visualization of soft tissue consistency, therefore delineating space-occupying lesions. Improved resolution of gray-scale instrumentation, together with high resolution real-time equipment, improves accuracy for diagnosis and localization of abscesses to approximately 95 percent. Ultrasound is a widely used modality for screening purposes and ^{67}Gallium scanning can also be used for screening; Gallium is particularly impressive for diagnosis of bone infections. However, in post operative patients uptake of ^{67}Gallium in the incision and gut frequently produces confusing appearances. In the diagnosis of inflammatory masses, one must differentiate between a phlegmon and an abscess. A *phlegmon* is an inflammatory solid mass which may resolve with or without treatment, or may proceed to form a fluid filled cavity containing pus, which is called an *abscess*. Surgical drainage is reserved for treatment of abscesses.

Clinical Symptoms

When a patient presents with malaise, fever of unknown origin, leukocytosis and shift to the left, with or without localizing signs, the possibility of an abdominal or pelvic inflammatory process with abscess formation must be considered. Gram-negative bacteria, in particular Escherichia coli, streptococci and staphylococci, are cultured. Clinical examination alone may lead to an early diagnosis such as in cases of appendicitis which would require immedi-

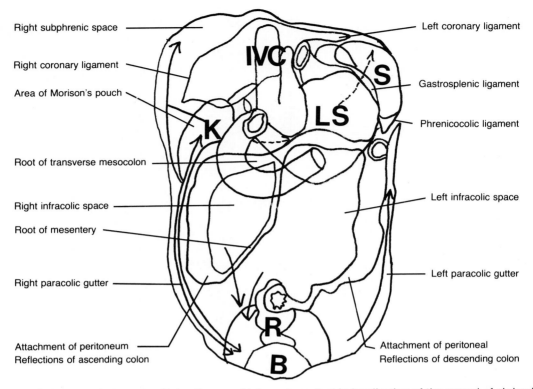

Fig. 11-1. Schema to show anatomical pathways which are important in localization of the spread of abdominal and pelvic abscesses. The root of the mesocolon divides the peritoneal cavity into a supracolic and infracolic compartment. Under the effects of gravity, pus can track down the paracolic gutter (solid arrows) into the pelvis or into the right subphrenic spaces. The dotted arrows indicate further possible spread anterior to the stomach into the left subphrenic space. (IVC = inferior vena cava, S = spleen, LS = lesser sac, K = right kidney, R = rectum, B = bladder).

ate surgery. However, more often, patients present with right upper quadrant tenderness and differential diagnosis includes acute cholecystitis, empyema of the gallbladder, subhepatic abscess or perinephric abscess. In the postoperative patient, fever may indicate a local wound abscess or spread of pus into the peritoneal or subhepatic spaces, or into the pelvis. Death may result from a delay in surgical drainage and antibiotic therapy.

Anatomic Sites for Abscesses

A thorough understanding of the anatomic pathways is necessary for localization of abdominal and pelvic abscesses. The important peritoneal spaces are delineated in Figures 11-1 and 11-2.

Intrahepatic Abscess While examining the liver with ultrasound, an intrahepatic abscess, subhepatic or subphrenic abscess may be found or multiple abscesses may be recognized. The presence of multiple abscesses will usually affect patient management; therefore if one abscess is found the liver should be carefully rescanned to exclude the possibility of multiple abscesses.

Liver abscesses may cause right upper quadrant pain but may have no localizing symptoms. The patient usually presents with fever of unknown origin, chills, pain and increased white blood cell count with a shift to the left. On ultrasound examination liver abscesses are generally sonolucent or echo free, and good through transmission is demonstrated posterior to the abscess. The normal liver

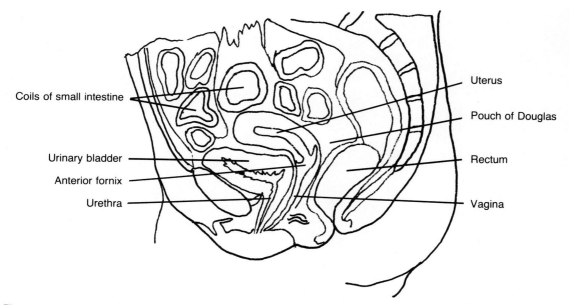

Fig. 11-2. Sagittal section of lower abdomen and pelvis in female. This demonstrates the relation of the pouch of Douglas to the uterus and rectum.

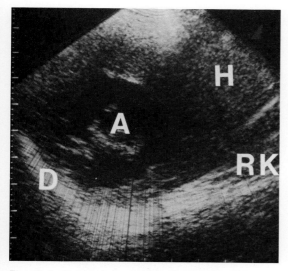

Fig. 11-3. Right subdiaphragmatic abscess. This appears as a large defect in the hepatic parenchyma (H). There is contained debris within the abscess (A). The diaphragm (D) is seen superiorly; the right kidney is seen inferiorly (RK).

tissue is echogenic and the patient may have hepatomegaly. An abscess, unlike a cyst, has irregular borders. Areas within the abscess may fill with debris (Fig. 11-3). After the ab-

scess is surgically drained, the physician may request follow up ultrasonic examinations to assess the patient's condition.

A chief cause for the formation of intrahepatic abscesses is organisms which attack the liver tissue through the bile ducts (ascending cholangitis), and blood borne infection through the hepatic artery and portal vein. Trauma is another cause for abscess formation in the liver.

Extrahepatic Abscess An extrahepatic abscess can occur in any of the potential spaces related to the peritoneal folds of the liver. The subphrenic or subdiaphragmatic space is a common site for these pus collections. This space is bordered by the diaphragm superiorly, by the abdominal wall posteriorly and by the abdominal wall anteriorly. The space continues to the transverse colon, but an abscess in this region involves the paracolic gutters. The right paracolic gutter is wide and deep and is continuous superiorly with the right subhepatic space and its postero-superior extension deep to the liver, which is surgically known as Morison's pouch (Fig. 11-4). The right subhepatic space is anatomically contin-

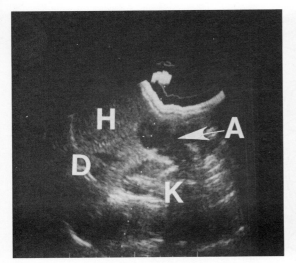

Fig. 11-4. Right subhepatic (anterior subphrenic) abscess cavity (A) in a neonate. The normal liver (H) is seen above the lesion and the right hemidiaphragm (D) is seen. The right kidney (K) is seen posteriorly.

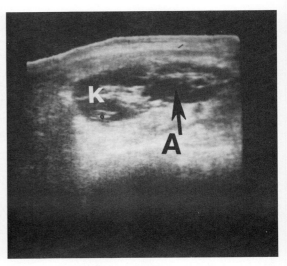

Fig. 11-5. Perinephric collection around a transplanted kidney in the left iliac fossa. The kidney (K) is seen on transverse section. A fluid collection (A) is seen medial to it. This could be a urinoma, lymphocele or abscess cavity. Drainage of pus demonstrated that this was an abscess.

uous with the right subphrenic space around the lateral edge of the right coronary ligament of the liver. The left paracolic gutter is narrow and shallow and is not continuous with the left subphrenic space.

Subphrenic Abscess Subphrenic and subhepatic abscesses are usually postoperative and are frequent following gastric operations and cholecystectomy. They are more common on the right side due to the proximity of the gallbladder, duodenum and appendix. The right subphrenic space is bordered by the diaphragm superiorly, and the liver inferiorly.

The left subphrenic space is bordered by the diaphragm superiorly, the left lobe of the liver posteriorly, and the anterior abdominal wall anteriorly. Pathology in the left kidney and spleen may cause pus formation in the left subphrenic space.

Renal Abscess A *renal abscess* may be referred to as a *renal carbuncle*. If a renal carbuncle ruptures it may cause a perirenal abscess, which has a sonolucent ultrasound appearance, often with an echogenic area within it (Fig. 11-5). Perirenal abscesses may also be due to infection or postoperative procedures.

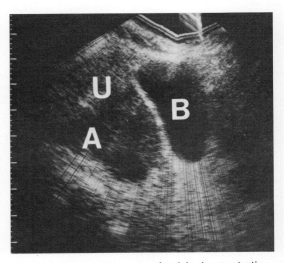

Fig. 11-6. Parasagittal scan of pelvis demonstrating a pelvic abscess. The bladder (B) is seen anteriorly and the uterus (U) is seen anterior to an ill defined fluid mass in the pouch of Douglas. These appearances are consistent with a pelvic abscess (A). Gut contents must be differentiated by repeat scanning or real-time scanning which demonstrates peristalsis.

Pelvic Abscess The pelvic peritoneum passes over the fundus of the uterus onto the posterior surface and is reflected onto the anterior surface of the rectum (p. 85). This forms the Pouch of Douglas and is a prime location for the development of pelvic abscesses.

The ultrasound characteristics of pelvic abscesses may be similar to those of complex pelvic masses such as endometriosis (Fig. 11-6). The most important factor in identifying an abscess is to differentiate the mass from the urinary bladder, uterus, ovaries and bowel (Fig. 11-7).

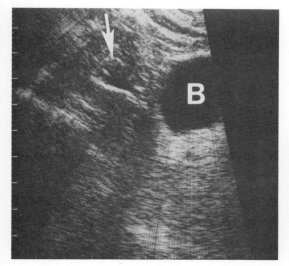

Fig. 11-7. Paramedian scan of the pelvis showing the bladder (B). A small fluid collection (arrowed) is seen superior to the bladder. This was not found to be constant on repeat scanning, and appearances are consistent with fluid in loops of bowel.

SCANNING TECHNIQUES

Mineral oil, or acoustical gel (on surgical sites) is applied to the abdominal skin surface. The highest frequency transducer possible is employed for best resolution; most often a 2.25 or 3.5 MHz transducer is appropriate for scanning the adult abdomen. The right upper abdomen is first examined in a series of parasagittal scans, beginning at the midline and scanning continuously to the outermost lateral portion of the body. Then transverse intercostal scans are obtained. The liver is used as an

acoustic window in the right upper quadrant. The same scanning technique described in p. 100 is again used for identifying a right upper quadrant abscess.

An abscess of the right upper quadrant can be successfully ruled out if the following regions are scanned carefully: the right subphrenic space, the entire intrahepatic region, the subhepatic space (Morison's pouch) and the right perinephric region. A longitudinal, single-sector scan allows visualization of the above regions in one plane (Fig. 11-8). With current gray-scale instrumentation, an abscess collection resembles a cystic, space-occupying lesion with internal echoes, representing debris. An area of high level echoes surrounding the abscess may be present. This represents inflammatory changes in the surrounding parenchyma.

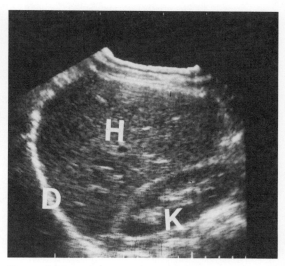

Fig. 11-8. Parasagittal scan through the right upper quadrant showing the normal liver (H), the right kidney (K) posteriorly and the right hemidiaphragm (D) superiorly. Multiple scans in the parasagittal plane allow confident exclusion of intrahepatic, subphrenic and subhepatic abscesses.

The left upper quadrant is usually examined best with the patient in the right decubitus position (left side up). The highest possible frequency transducer is used; a 3.5 MHz with narrow face (13 mm) is usually successful for intercostal scanning. The scanning arm is placed in the coronal plane of the midaxillary line; the transducer is placed in the lower intercostal spaces and angled cephalad. Small, single-sector scans are performed in this plane. This coronal technique which uses the spleen as an acoustic window is described in p. 158. Using this technique the left subphrenic space, left hemidiaphragm, spleen and the upper pole of the left kidney are clearly visualized (Fig. 11-9).

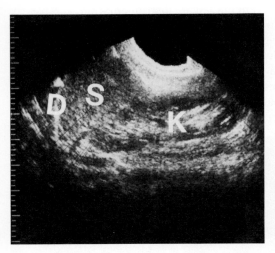

Fig. 11-9. Coronal scan of the left upper quadrant. The spleen (S) is used as an acoustic window to see the subphrenic space which is limited by the diaphragm (D) superiorly. The upper pole of the left kidney (K) is well seen.

The pelvis is scanned by using the distended urinary bladder as an acoustic window. With the bladder distended, the pouch of Douglas in the female and the rectovesical pouch in the male can be seen. Pelvic abscesses appear as fluid collections, spherical in shape, located in this pouch. Longitudinal and transverse scans are taken of the entire pelvis utilizing the technique described in pp. 85–86.

When fluid in the pelvis is present, the differential diagnosis must include: pelvic abscess, ovarian cyst and free ascites or fluid contained in loops of bowel. The ultrasonic criteria for the diagnosis of a pelvic abscess include: a rounded spherical contour, highly reflective, irregular walls and internal echoes

suggesting cellular debris contained in the pus. These ultrasound appearances, evaluated with the results of clinical examination and possibly a repeat ultrasound examination on the following day, result in an accurate diagnosis. There may be confusion between an ovarian cyst and a pelvic abscess, but ovarian cysts appear as round, thin walled lesions with few internal echoes. Septation of the cyst may be present. On clinical examination a pelvic abscess is a tender mass, fixed in position, while an ovarian cyst is mobile and usually nontender. Free ascites, which may also be seen in Morison's pouch, may be differentiated from abscess collections, as ascites will conform to adjacent organs in the intraperitoneal spaces, and changes in patient position will cause free ascites to move. Fluid filled loops of bowel usually appear as elongated structures. A repeat ultrasound examination the following day may show a noticeable change in the fluid filled bowel, while the abscess does not appear to change. High resolution real-time instrumentation is extremely helpful in differentiating bowel peristalsis from a pelvic abscess.

The midabdomen is scanned last, since it is a less common site for abdominal abscess. This region is also the most difficult and complex area to examine with ultrasound because

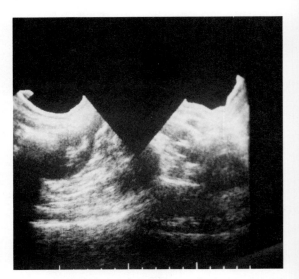

Fig. 11-10. Bilateral sector scans in the transverse plane of the left and right paracolic gutters.

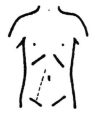

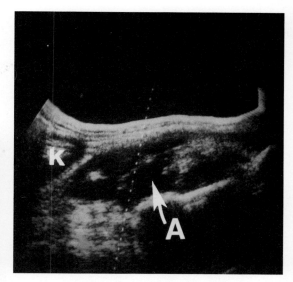

Fig. 11-12. Oblique longitudinal scan of the left paracolic gutter. There is a large, complex mass (A) from which a liter of pus was subsequently drained. The lower pole of the left kidney (K) can be seen above.

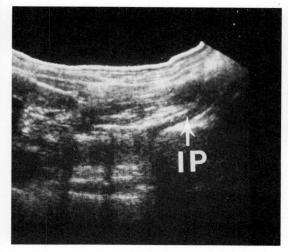

Fig. 11-11. Longitudinal oblique scan of the iliopsoas muscles (IP). The highly reflective structure seen in the middle of this muscle is probably the femoral nerve.

of overlying gut. The mechanical scanning arm is placed in the transverse position. Serial transverse sector scans are made bilaterally using the continuous survey mode. These short sector sweeps are produced by placing the transducer at the lateral portion of the midabdomen and sectoring towards the patient's midline. Scans are then repeated on the opposite side of the abdomen. (Fig. 11-10) Longitudinal scans of the midabdomen are obtained by passing the transducer rapidly down the anterior abdominal wall. The mechanical scanning arm is angled obliquely to allow scanning along the psoas muscles (Fig. 11-11). The iliac vessels, psoas muscles and paracolic gutters are well visualized along this axis. The midabdomen may be obscured by air-containing bowel, but if space-occupying masses are present, bowel is usually displaced and the mass well visualized (Fig. 11-12).

In conclusion, ultrasound is a widely used method for diagnosing and localizing abscesses, and is often used as a complementary study to [67]Gallium scanning. However, gallium studies may take several days to complete, and are often nonspecific. Ultrasound examination is performed quickly and is ideal for screening purposes.

SUGGESTED READING

Haaga JR, Alfidi RJ, Havrilla TR, Cooperman AM, et al: CT detection and aspiration of abdominal abscesses. AJR 128:465-474, 1977.

Meyers HA: The spread and localization of acute intra-peritoneal effusions. Radiology 95:547-554, 1970.

Taylor KJW, Moulton D: In Atlas of Gray-Scale Ultrasonography, ed. KJW Taylor, Edinburgh, Churchill Livingstone, 1978, pp 170-173.

Taylor KJW, Sullivan DC, Wasson JFMcI, Rosenfield AT: Ultrasound and gallium for the diagnosis of abdominal and pelvic abscesses. Gastrointestinal Radiol 3:281-286, 1978.

12

Spleen

CAROL A. TALMONT

INTRODUCTION

Ultrasound is a valuable modality for imaging the spleen since the spleen is a difficult organ to assess on physical examination due to its concealed position underneath the left costal margin. Before the spleen becomes palpable, it must be enlarged at least twice its normal size.

The spleen can be imaged by an isotope scan using ^{99m}Tc Sulphur colloid; space-occupying defects are revealed and an approximate splenic size is quantitated. Although computerized axial tomography is also used to evaluate splenic size and any defects of consistency, it does not differentiate between the various consistencies of the splenic parenchyma.

Ultrasound has been used to estimate the volume of the spleen since the introduction of bistable instrumentation. Gray-scale instrumentation displays the normal tissue consist-

ency, the presence of splenomegaly, and pathological tissue consistency. Using the techniques described in this chapter, the spleen may be visualized in all patients.

Anatomy and Physiology

The main functions of the spleen are to filter blood, break down red blood cells and provide an immune response. It is the largest organ of the reticuloendothelial system. The spleen is located in the left hypochondrial region, below the diaphragm, posterior and lateral to the stomach. The shape of the spleen is quite variable, but it has a relatively elongated body with a notched, anterior border. It is soft, extremely vascular and dark purple in color.

The spleen is covered by a capsule composed of fibrous elastic connective tissue, together with smooth muscle fibers. From the hilus, which is a fissure on the inferior surface, fibrous trabeculae spread into the organ. These offer support for the vessels and nerves which enter and leave the spleen at this point.

The blood supply of the spleen is derived from the splenic artery, the largest branch of the celiac axis. This large artery divides into six or more branches that enter the hilus and diverge in various directions throughout the splenic parenchyma. Each branch gives off smaller and smaller branches that deliver blood to sinusoids.

The splenic vein drains the spleen, and as it travels from the left to right toward the liver it is joined by the gastric, pancreatic and inferior mesenteric veins. The splenic vein then joins the superior mesenteric vein to form the portal vein posterior to the pancreatic neck.

Although the spleen is not essential to life, it does perform many important functions. In the fetus it is responsible for the production of red blood cells, but after delivery its functions are limited to the formation of lymphocytes, plasma cells and some monocytes. The phagocytic reticulo-endothelial cells of the spleen remove most of the old, worn out red blood cells from the circulatory system, taking iron from hemoglobin and recycling it into new red blood cells. Bilirubin links to protein, enters the blood stream (indirect reacting bilirubin pp. 112 – 114), and is carried to the liver for conversion to water soluble glucuronides (direct reacting bilirubin) before secretion into the bile. The spleen produces plasma cells and antibodies, that aid in the protection against various diseases and viruses. Realization of these important immunologic functions has made splenectomy undesirable, especially in children.

SCANNING TECHNIQUES

The anatomy of the spleen shows many normal variations. The sonographer should always be aware of these normal variations when scanning the organ to identify normal vascular structures.

For optimal visualization of the entire spleen, the patient is placed in the right lateral decubitus position (left side up). The patient's arm should be abducted over the head to widen the intercostal spaces (Fig. 12-1). Ultrasonic gel provides an excellent coupling agent since it can be heavily applied and used as a cushion between the ribs and transducer face. A rolled towel may be placed under the patient's right side (midabdomen) to reduce the iliac curve. This gives increased mobility when sectoring the spleen.

The spleen is only rarely delineated by ultrasound with the patient in the supine position. Indeed, if the spleen is visualized in the parasagittal plane, splenomegaly must be suspected.

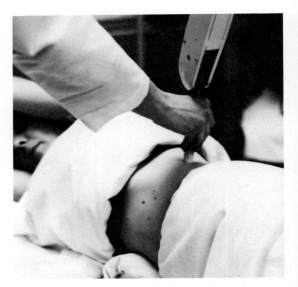

Fig. 12-1. Coronal plane used for longitudinal spleen scan, with the patient in the right decubitus position.

With the patient in the right lateral decubitus position, the scanning arm is placed in the longitudinal position along the patient's midaxillary line. Coronal scans are obtained simply by angling the transducer underneath the costal margin towards the patient's head, to produce a single sector sweep in the caudad direction. It is most beneficial if the patient inspires, to depress the left hemidiaphragm. The left portion of the diaphragm, the superior border of the spleen, and the left kidney are visualized on one coronal scan. Since ultrasound is a tomographic technique, the spleen

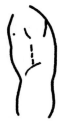

Front

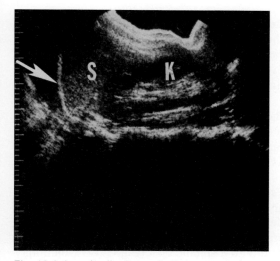

Fig. 12-2. Longitudinal scan in the coronal plane, showing the left kidney (K), the spleen (S) and the left hemidiaphragm (arrowed).

should be scanned from the most posterior section to the most anterior part of the organ using the continuous survey mode. By this time, the examiner will have obtained a mental, three-dimensional picture of the size, shape and consistency of the organ. It is the sonographer's responsibility to examine approximately 50 sections of the spleen in the coronal plane, but to record only approximately three scans on hard copy with pertinent information (Fig. 12-2).

After thoroughly examining the spleen in the coronal plane from the posterior to anterior portion, the oblique plane is then approached. The patient remains in the right lateral decubitus position. The mechanical scanning arm is moved behind the patient and angled parallel to the lower left intercostal spaces, so that the spleen can be scanned sub-

costally and intercostally (Fig. 12-3). The sonographer then starts with the superior section of the spleen slightly inferior to the left hemidiaphragm. The patient is asked to inspire and hold respiration while a sector scan is performed from the anterior aspect of the patient to the posterior aspect in one single sector sweep (Fig. 12-4). The sonographer proceeds to scan inferiorly using various intercostal spaces. It may be possible to examine the entire organ subcostally in varying degrees of respiration by using the oblique plane. The spleen is visualized from the most superior border to the most inferior lobe. The upper pole of the left kidney is delineated in cross-section quite clearly in this plane. Angling the transducer cephalad allows a greater portion of the spleen to be visualized. Using this technique avoids scanning over the ribs which produce shadowing artifacts.

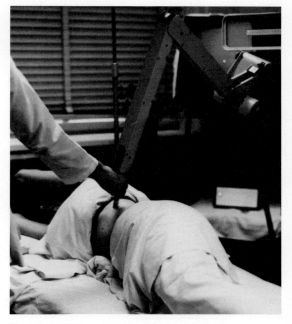

Fig. 12-3. Oblique intercostal scan along the long axis of the spleen.

Serial oblique scans have proved successful in evaluating splenic volume and estimating the weight of the organ. Generally the normal spleen returns low-level echoes. The TGC is adjusted to produce an even distribution of these echoes throughout the splenic

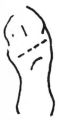

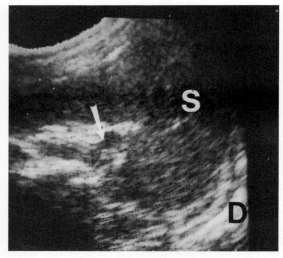

Fig. 12-4. Oblique intercostal scan of the spleen (S). The vessels leaving the hilum of the spleen are arrowed. D = left hemidiaphragm.

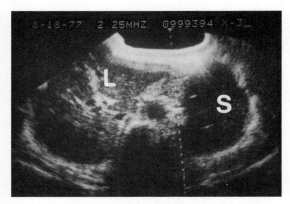

Fig. 12-5. Transverse scan of abdomen showing marked splenomegaly (S). Note that the amplitude of the echoes is considerably lower than that from the liver substance (L).

parenchyma. Recent studies indicate that no specific patterns are associated exclusively with any particular pathology. However, patients with untreated malignant lymphoma or leukemia usually have enlarged, black spleens (low-level echoes) (Fig. 12-5). Splenomegaly due to portal hypertension presents a fine echo pattern of medium amplitude throughout the spleen and splenomegaly due to inflammatory causes returns high level echoes.

PATHOLOGY

Congenital Anomalies Congenital absence of the spleen (asplenia; agenesis of the spleen) is rare and causes no complications alone. However, asplenia is often associated with congenital heart disease (Fig. 12-6).

A more common congenital anomaly is the presence of accessory spleens, most often located in the tail of the pancreas. Lesions may occur in these accessory spleens as well as in the main organ.

Focal Defects Focal defects of the spleen are apparent on radioisotope scanning and patients are referred to ultrasound for differentiation as to the cause. Such focal defects may be due to a splenic cyst (Fig. 12-7) which may be congenital, traumatic or parasitic in origin. Focal metastatic tumor involvement of the spleen is rare, with the exception of melanoma and lymphoma. Generally, metastases to the spleen appear highly echogenic, but focal lymphoma involvement usually produces hypo-echoic lesions. However, lymphoma of the spleen is generally more diffuse, and results in splenomegaly with lower echo amplitude than the normal splenic parenchyma.

Infarcts are areas of tissue death caused by occlusion of the splenic artery or its smaller branches. They often occur due to emboli thrown from infected material on the heart valves (bacterial endocarditis, a disease now widely seen in drug addicts). The ultrasonic appearances of infarcts vary according to the time since onset. A newly formed hemorrhagic infarct appears more sonolucent than normal splenic tissue. As organization occurs with the formation of scar tissue, an echogenic lesion is formed, characteristically triangular in shape with the base towards the surface of the organ (Fig. 12-8).

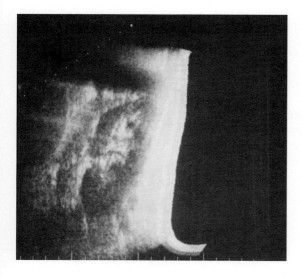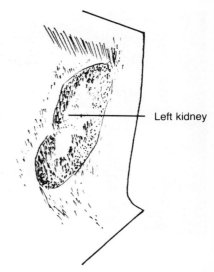

Fig. 12-6. Longitudinal scan showing the left kidney. There is no evidence of the spleen in this patient with asplenia. The patient is in the upright position.

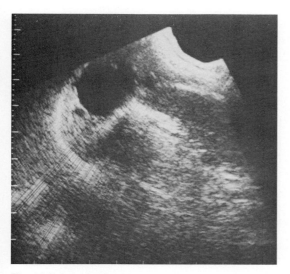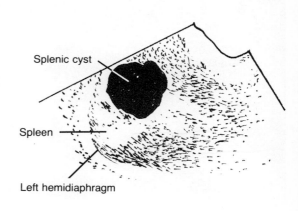

Fig. 12-7. Longitudinal scan of the spleen in the coronal plane. An echo-free area is seen within the spleen, consistent with a splenic cyst.

Splenomegaly The longitudinal axis of the normal spleen measures 10 cm, and must be regarded as pathologically enlarged if this measurement exceeds 12 cm. Characteristically, portal hypertension, the most common cause of splenomegaly in this country, shows enlargement of the spleen between 12 to 20 cm, and there is a fine echo pattern of medium amplitude throughout the organ (Fig. 12-9).

There is often other evidence of portal hypertension, such as an enlarged, tortuous splenic and portal vein. Splenomegaly may also be due to inflammatory causes such as tuberculosis, mononucleosis, malaria and sarcoidosis, which return high level echoes. The size of the spleen gives some indication of the possible underlying pathology. Various causes of splenomegaly are listed in Table 12-1.

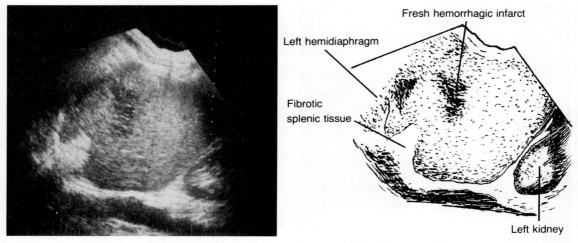

Fig. 12-8. Longitudinal scan of the spleen in the coronal plane. A recent hemorrhagic infarct is shown, and an older infarct is seen near the diaphragmatic surface.

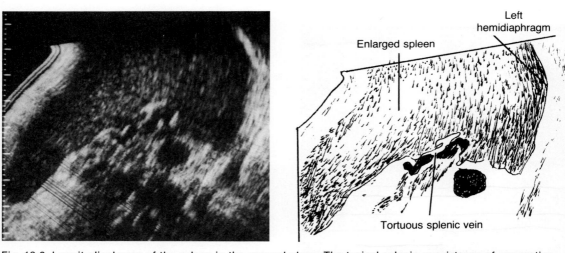

Fig. 12-9. Longitudinal scan of the spleen in the coronal plane. The typical splenic consistency of congestive splenomegaly is seen. Multiple branches of the splenic vein are seen leaving the hilum of the spleen.

TABLE 12-1. VARIOUS CAUSES OF SPLENOMEGALY

A. Massive Splenomegaly (over 1000 gm)
   chronic myelogenous leukemia
   chronic lymphocytic leukemia (less massive)
   lymphomas
   myeloid metaplasia
   malaria
   Gaucher's Disease
   primary tumors of the spleen (rare)
B. Moderate Splenomegaly (500-1000 gm)
   chronic congestive splenomegaly (portal vein or
      splenic vein obstruction)
   infectious mononucleosis
   acute leukemia
   early sickle cell anemia
   hereditary spherocytosis
   thalassemia
   autoimmune hemolytic anemia
   idiopathic thrombocytopenic purpura
   Niemann - Pick Disease
   Hand - Schuller - Christian Disease
   chronic splenitis (vegetative endocarditis)
   tuberculosis, sarcoidosis, typhoid
   metastatic carcinoma or sarcoma
C. Minimal Splenomegaly (150-500 gm)
   acute splenitis
   acute splenic congestion

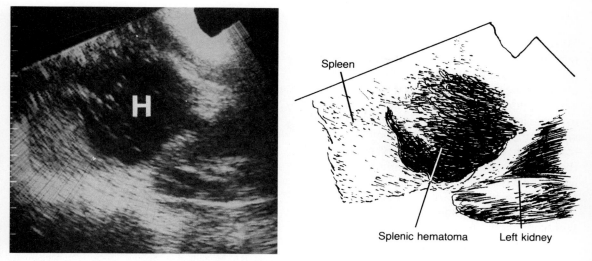

Fig. 12-10. Longitudinal scan of the spleen in the coronal plane. A large homogeneous space-occupying mass is seen within the splenic substance. This proved to be a large hematoma (H).

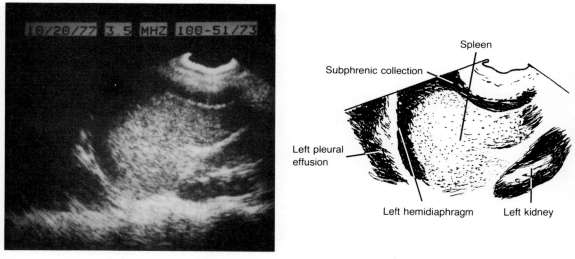

Fig. 12-11. Longitudinal scan of the spleen in the coronal plane. An echogenic spleen is seen in a splenic phlegmon with a surrounding subphrenic collection.

Rupture of the Spleen The normal spleen may rupture as a result of trauma to the left side of the chest (such as that incurred in automobile accidents). In addition, an enlarged, soft spleen, often found in infectious mononucleosis, malaria, leukemia or typhoid fever, may rupture spontaneously. Rupture of the spleen is a life-threatening condition if there is extensive bleeding into the peritoneal cavity.

A hematoma around the spleen (Fig. 12-10) must be differentiated from a subphrenic abscess (Fig. 12-11). In practice, this differentiation is entirely a clinical one. The patient with a subphrenic abscess usually presents with fever, high white blood cell count and shift to the left. The patient with a hematoma gives a history of trauma, and symptoms of blood loss such as faintness and hypotension.

CONCLUSION

Ultrasound scanning of the left upper quadrant provides valuable information on the size and parenchymal consistency of the spleen. In addition, the spleen can be used as an acoustic window into the left upper quadrant, and allows the left subphrenic space, the left adrenal and the upper pole of the left kidney to be well imaged. In view of the difficulty reported in the literature in diagnosing pathology in the left upper quadrant, the decubitus position appears to be particularly satisfactory for visualization of the spleen and surrounding pathology.

SUGGESTED READING

Bhimji SD, Cooperberg PL, Naiman S, Morrison RT, Shergill P: Ultrasound diagnosis of splenic cysts. Radiology 122:787-789, 1977.

de Graaff CS, Taylor KJW, Jacobson P: Grey scale echography of the spleen: follow-up in 67 patients. Ultrasound Med Biol 5:13-23, 1979.

Gordon DH, Burrell MI, Levin DC, Mueller CR, Becker JA: Wandering spleen—the radiological and clinical spectrum. Radiology 125:39-46, 1977.

Hunter TB, Haber K: Sonographic diagnosis of a wandering spleen. AJR 129:925-926, 1977.

Taylor KJW: Ultrasonic investigation of the hepatobiliary system and spleen. In: Ultrasonics in Clinical Diagnosis, 2nd Ed, ed. Wells PNT. Edinburgh, Churchill Livingstone, 1977.

Taylor KJW, Milan J: Differential diagnosis of chronic splenomegaly by grey-scale ultrasonography: Clincal observation and digital A-scan analysis. Br J Radiol 49:519-525, 1976.

Taylor KJW, Moulton D: The spleen. In: Atlas of Gray Scale Ultrasonography, ed. Taylor KJW. Edinburgh, Churchill Livingston, 1978.

Tuttle RJ, Minielly JA: Splenic cystic lymphangiomatosis: An unusual cause of massive splenomegaly. Radiology 126:47-48, 1978.

13

Adrenal Glands

CAROL A. TALMONT

INTRODUCTION

In the past, the adrenal glands were rarely visualized with ultrasound due to instrument limitations. Now, with the development of sophisticated gray-scale instrumentation, diffuse differences in parenchyma are appreciated. In addition, the current use of focused transducers has greatly improved lateral resolution. With the improved technical expertise in examining the adrenals, a success rate of 85 percent visualization has been achieved in patients studied by Sample in 1977.

Anatomy

The adrenal glands are located superior to the upper pole of the kidneys. They are essential for life and responsible for a wide variety of endocrine activities. Two different parts of the gland are recognized, the medulla and the cor-

tex, each having markedly different functions and embryologic derivation.

The anatomy of each of the adrenal glands varies and is shown schematically in Figure 13-1. The right adrenal is shaped like a cocked hat sitting on the top of the right kidney; the left adrenal is crescentic and extends down the superior-medial aspect. Each gland is approximately 5.0 cm long, 3.0 cm wide and 1.0 cm in the anterior-posterior plane. In the normal patient, the glands are surrounded by variable amounts of perirenal fat, which makes their precise delineation difficult. On cut sections, the gland is seen to consist of an outer layer (cortex) and an inner area (medulla). To date, separation of the cortex and medulla by gray-scale ultrasound has not been successful.

Physiology

The cortex of the adrenal is an endocrine gland which secretes three types of hormones.

165

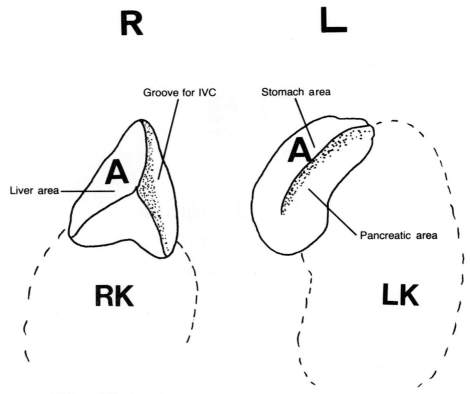

Fig. 13-1. Schema to show shape of adrenal glands (A) and their relation to the kidneys. The right adrenal gland is triangular in outline and surmounts the upper pole of the right kidney (RK). The left adrenal is crescentic and covers the superior and medial borders of the left kidney (LK).

(1) The glucocorticoids, of which cortisone and hydrocortisone are the most important. These hormones regulate carbohydrate metabolism, are important in the response to stress, and are essential for the maintenance of normal blood pressure. (2) The mineralcorticoids, the most important of which is aldosterone, control sodium excretion by the kidney and are directly responsible for the maintenance of normal body fluid balance. In the absence of aldosterone, body water is lost resulting in the inability to maintain blood pressure, and leading to early death. (3) Androgens, and to a lesser extent estrogens, are also secreted. Although androgens are principally produced in the testes in the male, and estrogens by the ovaries in the female, the opposite sex hormone is secreted in appreciable quantities by the adrenal, and this is important for normal sexual activity.

The secretion of all these hormones is under control of the pituitary (hypophysis cerebri), which is in turn under the control of the hypothalmus, situated in the base of the brain.

The adrenal medulla is composed of two types of cells, one neural in origin, and the other endocrine. Because of their staining property with bichromic acid, the nerve cells are called pheochromocytes. These cells secrete adrenalin and are an important part of the sympathetic nervous system. Stimulation of the sympathetic nervous system causes the release of adrenalin, which results in the typical changes associated with fear and excitement, namely increased heart rate, increased blood pressure, pallor of the skin and sweating. However, in daily activity the sympathetic system is predominantly responsible for blood vessel tone, which allows the maintenence of blood pressure despite changes in posture.

Imaging of the Adrenal Glands

Until the advent of the gray-scale ultrasonography, the adrenal glands were difficult to image by any radiological method. Introduction of air into the peritoneum was utilized to outline the adrenal glands which are retroperitoneal structures. Where available, computerized axial tomography is now technically the easiest way to display the normal adrenal glands, since the normal glands are not easily displayed by ultrasound. However, we have successfully used ultrasound to display cysts, adenomas and malignant tumors arising from the adrenal glands. The sonographer must use proper gain application to appreciate the few low-level echoes within a mass. This is necessary to evaluate whether an adrenal mass is cystic or solid and is sometimes critical in diagnosing the type of tumor. The adrenal glands can be scanned with the kidneys, and a new approach has been described by Sample using the decubitus position and precise anatomical alignment with known landmarks.

ULTRASOUND SCANNING TECHNIQUES

The key factor in successfully scanning the adrenal glands is the precise alignment between the left kidney and the aorta and between the right kidney and the inferior vena cava. Both adrenals are situated between the kidneys and these great vessels. The valsalva maneuver is not essential in examining the right adrenal gland. The exact coronal (longitudinal) scanning plane is determined by the following technique: transverse scans are carried out at the level of the lower, mid- and upper portions of the kidney, and the midaxis of the kidney is marked on the patient's skin. A point is also marked on the patient's body which will show the relationship between the center of the kidney and the aorta (Fig. 13-2A). From these plotted points obtained on the transverse scans, the longitudinal oblique scanning plane is determined. The axis of the scanning plane is oblique because the lower pole of the kidney is situated more anterior than the upper pole. Scans are obtained along this longitudinal oblique axis. The angle of the scanning plane is established from the transverse scan, considering the relationship of the upper pole of the kidney to the great vessel. A slight anterior angulation may be necessary for adequate scans. The sonographer may also scan parallel to the longitudinal plane established, and the degree of angulation may be varied. However, the oblique axis of the plane described previously from the transverse scans should not be changed.

Scans obtained utilizing this approach demonstrate the aorta, the left kidney and the spleen, or the inferior vena cava, the right kidney and the liver (Fig. 13-2 A – C). The area between the three structures on the left or right side represents either the left or right adrenal gland. Due to the echogenic nature of both the gland and the perirenal fat, it may be difficult to separate the adrenal gland from this fatty tissue.

The sonographer should ask the patient to suspend respiration to prevent artifacts resembling adrenal masses. Another artifact encountered in adrenal ultrasonography is the shadowing from the overlying rib cage. Both of these artifacts can be avoided by using a transducer with a small face, such as 13 mm diameter. Such a transducer, at a frequency of 3.5 MHz, can be rocked in the lower intercostal spaces and produce a small sector scan. Figures 13-3 and 13-4 show scans of the normal adrenal glands obtained by the techniques described above. Note that the medulla and cortex are not differentiated by ultrasound with currently available signal processing.

PATHOLOGY

Adrenal masses may be delineated either above or medial to the kidney. Ultrasound can identify these lesions and determine their solid or cystic nature (Fig. 13-5). Calcification produces very high level echoes with an occasional posterior acoustic shadow.

Pathology of the adrenals is related to the tumors arising from them, and their under- or over-production of hormones. Tumors

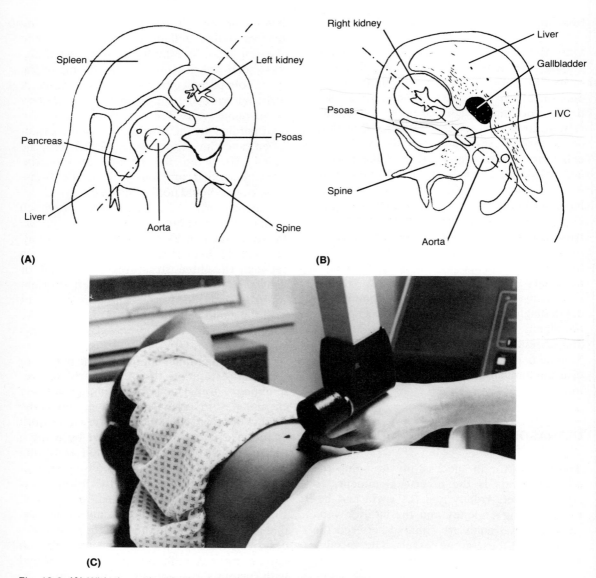

Fig. 13-2. **(A)** With the patient in the right decubitus position (left side up), the plane of the left kidney is marked on the skin surface. The scanning plane to the left adrenal now lies between the midplane of the left kidney and the aorta. **(B)** With the patient in the left decubitus position (right side up), the plane of the right adrenal gland lies between the midpoint of the right kidney and the inferior vena cava. **(C)** Photography to show the position of the scanning arm for scanning the right adrenal gland using the technique described in **(B)**.

whether benign or malignant, may secrete hormones in excess and produce well-recognized clinical syndromes. Endocrine deficiencies may be produced when the gland is destroyed by hemorrhage, infarction or tumor. In view of the control of the adrenals by the pituitary, excess and insufficiency states may also be produced by pituitary dysfunction.

The following are cortical syndromes.

Waterhouse-Fridericksen Syndrome is most commonly due to bilateral hemorrhage into the adrenal glands, usually due to an overwhelming septic state. Hemorrhagic destruction of the adrenals may be found on scanning. Patients with this syndrome are acutely ill and unable to maintain blood pressure. Pro-

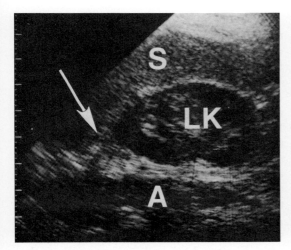

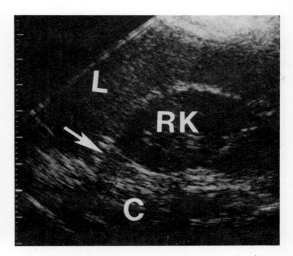

Fig. 13-3. Scan obtained using the technique described in Figure 13-2A showing the aorta (A), spleen (S), left kidney (KL) and the normal left adrenal (arrowed).

Fig. 13-4. Scan of the right adrenal obtained using the technique described in Fig. 13-2B.

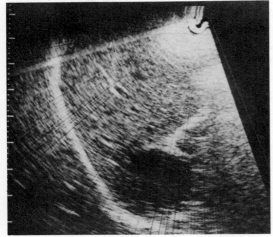

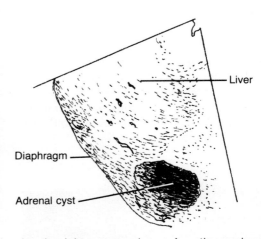

Fig. 13-5. Parasagittal scan through intercostal space showing the right suprarenal area. A cystic area is seen in the right suprarenal position consistent with an adrenal cyst.

nounced hypotension occurs in the course of a fulminating septic state, and cortisone therapy is life-saving.

Addison's Disease may be adrenal or pituitary in origin and is the chronic result of hypofunction of the adrenal glands, characterized by dysfunction of carbohydrate and endocrine metabolism and hypotension. Adrenal deficiency may be due to a primary tumor or metastases in the adrenals; lung tumors frequently metastasize to the adrenals.

Cushing's Syndrome is produced by excessive secretion of glucocorticoids, usually due to hyperplasia of the adrenal cortex but occasionally due to a benign tumor (adenoma, Fig. 13-6) and more rarely due to a carcinoma. Alternatively, this syndrome can be produced by a tumor from the anterior pituitary. The syndrome consists of obesity, hirsuitism, sexual impotence and hypertension. The face is characteristically moon-shaped and purple, with acne and purple lines like exaggerated stretchmarks.

Conn's Syndrome is caused by excessive secretion of aldosterone, usually by a

*neuroblastoma – Ca adre[n]
in children*

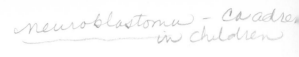

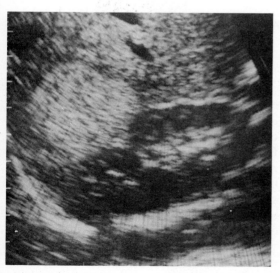

Fig. 13-6. Adrenal scan obtained using the technique described in Fig. 13-2A. The spleen (S) is seen above the left kidney (LK). The aorta (A) is seen posteriorly. A solid adrenal mass (a) is seen, consistent with an adrenal adenoma.

cortical adenoma and results in abnormal retention of sodium with hypertension.

Adreno-genital Syndrome is due to excessive secretion of the sex hormones, which produce virilism in the female and early sexual development in the male.

The two types of cells in the adrenal medulla give rise to different clinical syndromes. The pheochromocytes may produce a tumor, (pheochromocytoma) which secretes adrenalin and noradrenalin in excessive quantities. Such patients present with intermittent hypertension. The patient shown in Figure 13-7 had intractable hypertension for three years, and pheochromocytoma was diagnosed initially by ultrasound. The patient nearly died immediately before surgery owing to uncontrollable hypertension, demonstrating the need for early diagnosis of such lesions. Arteriography is hazardous in such patients since this may provoke a hypertensive episode. Figure 13-8A and B show another adrenal pheochromocytoma presenting as a right adrenal mass with a necrotic center. Note the mass compressing the inferior vena cava. This patient was a 52-year-old woman with history of high blood pressure and abnormally high cortisone levels. Angiography had demonstrated a vascular right adrenal mass.

CONCLUSION

Gray-scale ultrasonography of the adrenals is a new technique which was first described by

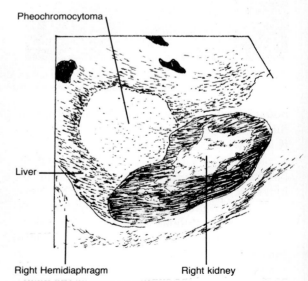

Fig. 13-7. Parasagittal scan of a 27 year-old patient with intractable hypertension. A suprarenal mass 5 cm in diameter is seen above the right kidney. Subsequent exploration revealed a pheochromocytoma.

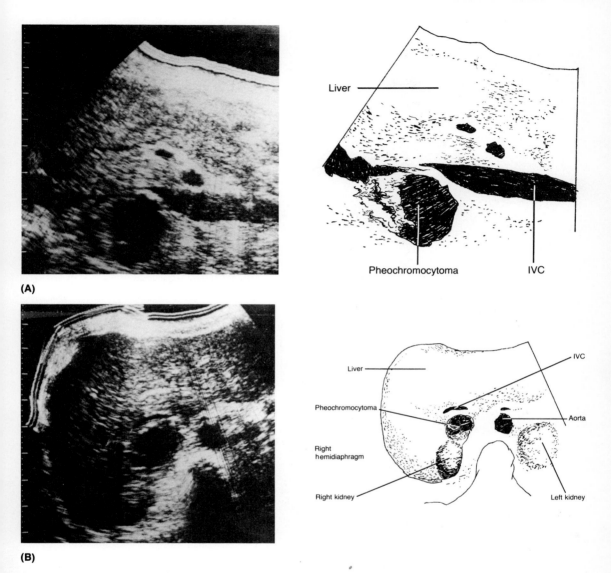

(A)

(B)

Fig. 13-8. **(A)** Longitudinal scan in the plane of the inferior vena cava. A large, partially necrotic mass, is seen posterior to the inferior vena cava in the right suprarenal position. **(B)** Transverse scan showing a predominantly cystic lesion posterior to the inferior vena cava. This cystic lesion compresses the lumen of the inferior vena cava. These appearances are consistent with a cystic necrotic mass, derived from the adrenal gland. This mass proved to be a pheochromocytoma.

Sample in 1977. Before that time, only large masses and cysts were delineated, mainly on the right side, where the use of the liver as an acoustic window makes a more conventional approach to the right suprarenal area possible. The use of flexible scanning techniques should be stressed, and the supine as well as the decubitus positions for scanning in the midaxillary plane can be used in addition to the specialized procedures described to scan the adrenals.

SUGGESTED READING

Sample WF: A new technique for the evaluation of the adrenal gland with gray-scale ultrasonography. Radiology 124:463-469, 1977.

14

Biopsy and Aspiration Technique

RALPH WINTERS

INTRODUCTION

Although ultrasound is regarded as the least invasive imaging modality, at this institution and at many others, it is increasingly being used in conjunction with invasive diagnostic methods. No patient need undergo repeated, unsuccessful attempts at chest aspiration to investigate the cause of an opacity on a chest X-ray when ultrasound can not only demonstrate whether the opacity is due to fluid or a solid lesion, but also indicates the optimal site for successful aspiration. In other patients, aspiration of renal cysts allows the exclusion of malignancy while ultrasonically guided liver biopsy with a skinny needle or cutting needle frequently makes an exploratory laparotomy unnecessary. This increasing invasion of the body under ultrasound guidance puts new responsibilities on the sonographer, if these

minor surgical procedures are to be undertaken in safety.

Responsibilities of the Sonographer

The sonographer working in an invasive laboratory must have a thorough knowledge of possible complications that could arise during any procedure. A CPR cart should be available in case of sudden emergencies. It is the sonographer's responsibility to see that all biopsies and aspirations are done in accordance with the principles of good surgical aseptic technique. There is danger of infection and contamination when many of these minor surgical procedures are performed, and it may be necessary to carry out disinfection of the room. The scanning arm and the transducer, as well as any hand-held controls, should be cleaned especially well.

It is also the sonographer's responsibility to ensure that appropriate trays are ready for the physician who will perform the procedure. The choice of needles should be established in advance and the suitable variety of needles and surgical gloves provided.

If doughnut or slot transducers are employed, they must be sent for gas sterilization. This is a slow procedure requiring up to 72 hours, so scheduling of patients should be done well in advance. The sonographer must be familiar with the tests to which the aspirate will be submitted and have the appropriate requisition slips available. Finally, the sonographer is responsible for ensuring that the consent form has been signed before the procedure commences, and that results of all blood work are available for the physician.

The sonographer plays a strong supportive role towards the patient during these procedures. Most of these procedures are innocuous but are nevertheless feared by patients, who require reassurance. Occasionally a patient may feel faint. If the patient is pregnant, this is usually due to pressure on the inferior vena cava occluding blood return to the heart and should be treated by turning the patient on her side. In nonpregnant patients the faintness may be due to anxiety, provoking a vasovagal attack. The head should be lowered and, if recovery is not immediate, blood pressure and pulse should be monitored by a nurse or physician.

Following an invasive procedure, the patient should be allowed to rest under observation for a period of time. After amniocentesis this may be only 30 minutes, while patients who have had deep biopsies, for example of the pancreas, should be observed for 6 hours. All patients should be checked by a physician before leaving the department.

THORACENTESIS UNDER ULTRASONIC GUIDANCE

Anatomy The thorax comprises the upper portion of the torso and contains the heart and lungs. It is limited below by the diaphragm and above by the thoracic inlet. The thoracic cavity is bounded by the spine and ribs posteriorly and by the sternum, costal cartilage and ribs anteriorly. Classically, the thorax is divided into the lung fields, the heart and great vessels. The right and left lung fields are comprised of three and two lobes respectively. The mediastinum (the area between the lungs) is subidivided into the superior and inferior portions by a line which passes horizontally through the second costal cartilage. This level can be quickly identified by running the fingers down the front of the sternum. Approximately two inches from the top of the sternum (the manubrium) is a definite deflection known as the angle of Louis. This is the junction of the manubrium and the body of the sternum, and a horizontal line at this level intersects the body of the fourth thoracic vertebra. Above this plane is the superior mediastinum which contains the great vessels, and, in particular, the arch of the aorta with its branches, the superior vena cava and brachiocephalic veins. Below this plane the inferior mediastinum contains the heart in the space between the medial aspects of the lungs, and posterior to the heart, those tubes which transmit to and from the thoracic cavity. These include the esophagus, trachea, great veins and great arteries.

The lungs are surrounded by a thin, double layered membrane, the pleura. The arrangement of the pleura can be visualized as a lung bud growing into a structure like a balloon. As the lung bud grows, it invaginates itself into the balloon as shown in Figure 14-1A to C, and eventually becomes completely enclosed by two layers of membrane. These layers of pleura normally have only a very small amount of fluid between them, which reduces friction as the lungs collapse and expand during respiration. This arrangement is similar to systems that exist around the heart (pericardium), the bowel (peritoneum) and around the tendon sheaths (synovium). A pleural effusion is a collection of fluid which distends and fills this sac (Fig. 14-1D).

Ultrasound examination of the aerated lungs is impossible due to the major difference in acoustical impedance between soft tissue and air, which results in virtually total reflec-

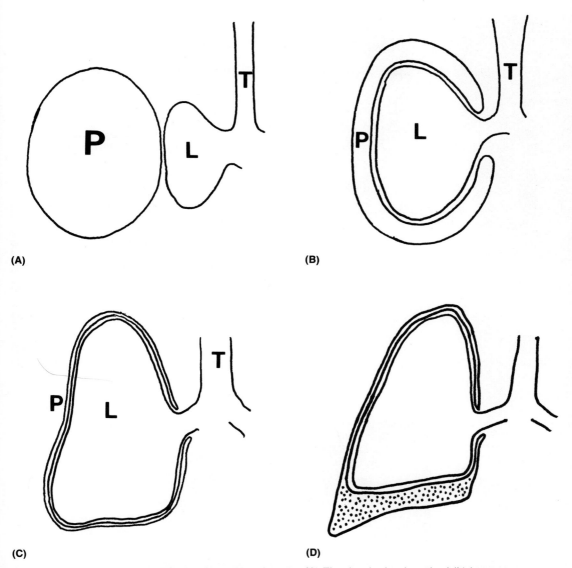

Fig. 14-1. Schema to show anatomy of the pleural space. **(A)** The developing lung bud (L) becomes approximated to the pleural sac (P). T = Trachea. **(B)** The growing bud is invaginated into the pleural space, which becomes stretched around it as a double layer. **(C)** Final arrangement of the pleura is a double layer, completely surrounding the lung. In the normal patient there is virtually no separation between the layers of the pleura, so that the pleural cavity is a potential space. **(D)** When fluid accumulates between the layers of the pleura, the layers separate and the pleural effusion causes compression and collapse of the lung above it.

tion of the ultrasound beam. However, when there is fluid in the chest, ultrasound examination becomes useful, particularly in differentiating between solid and fluid consistencies. Routine chest radiographs show an opaque appearance for both consolidation of the lung and pleural effusion. The presence of fluid may be deduced from decubitus films which may show layering with gravity. When an effusion is encapsulated, however, and not free to move with gravity, this layering does not occur and pleural effusions then become

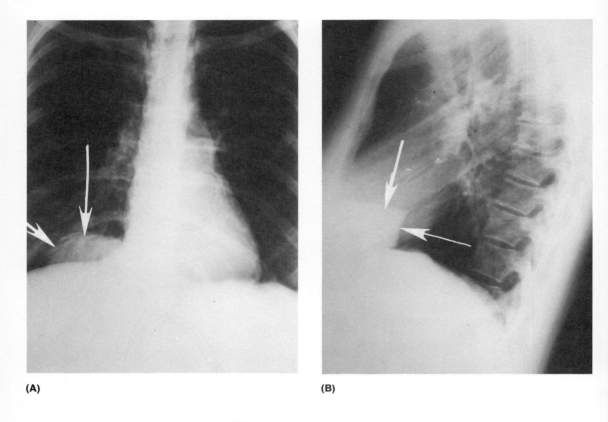

(A)

(B)

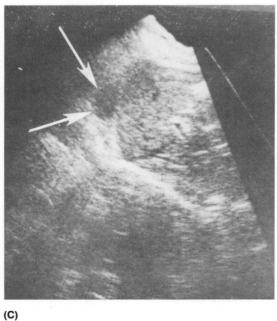

(C)

Fig. 14-2. **(A)** Posteroanterior radiograph showing opacity in right lower lobe (arrowed). **(B)** Lateral radiograph showing right lower lobe opacity (arrowed). **(C)** Ultrasound examination shows a complex lesion (arrowed) above the right hemidiaphragm which is not a simple fluid collection.

difficult to evaluate using standard radiographic techniques. Under these circumstances, ultrasound is an excellent modality to evaluate radio-opaque masses in the thorax further. Figures 14-2A and B are posteroanterior and lateral chest radiographs showing a right lower lobe opacity. The ultrasound scan (Fig. 14-2C) shows that this is not a simple effusion.

Technique The thoracic cavity may need to be aspirated under ultrasound guidance if a blind thoracocentesis has been unsuccessful. Usually the medical or surgical residents perform the tap on the information provided by the sonographer. In difficult cases the ultrasonologist supervises the procedure. At this institution neither the doughnut nor the slot transducer are routinely used in chest aspirations; we find it easier to identify an appropriate area for aspiration and then to remove all ultrasound apparatus and tap the chest either in the ultrasound laboratory or on the ward. In addition to aspirating cystic collections, an intrathoracic tumor may be localized for biopsy under ultrasound guidance (Fig. 14-3).

Prior to the actual aspiration procedure, the exact position of the fluid should be identified with the patient in different positions. Recent PA and lateral chest X-rays are helpful in showing the optimal position to begin scanning. If the right side of the chest is opaque, the patient can be scanned in the supine position, using the liver as an acoustic window as in a routine liver scan (Fig. 14-4A). A parasagittal scan may show free fluid above the diaphragm in the costophrenic angle. The fluid nature of the collection must be confirmed by observing the A-scans. While the actual aspiration is not performed in the supine position, scanning from the medial to lateral direction through the subcostal and intercostal spaces gives a rapid overall indication of the location and extent of a right pleural effusion. A left pleural effusion is approached initially in the right decubitus position (left side up) using the spleen as an acoustic window (pp. 158–159), and scanning the area above and below the left hemidiaphragm (Fig. 14-4B).

After these preliminary scans are completed, the patient adopts an upright position, sitting on the edge of the stretcher. The fluid is again localized by scanning in the intercostal spaces from the posterior aspect (Fig. 14-5). The right and left chest give similar pictures in the upright position (Fig. 14-6A and B). Multiple scans should be performed in deep inspiration, expiration and during normal quiet breathing to assess the true mobility of the area of interest. This also gives an accurate assessment of diaphragmatic movement. At this time, the chest may be tapped, or the position of the fluid marked on the skin surface and the patient returned to the ward for aspiration there. If the patient is tapped in the ultrasound section, a post-aspiration scan should be obtained (Fig. 14-7A and B).

Skin pencils are generally unsatisfactory for marking the position of the fluid collection, since they are usually removed during sterilization. When aspiration is performed immediately after localization with ultrasound, we use an imprint on the skin from the hub of a needle as a marker. An alternative technique is to provide two arrows outside the field of sterilization which, when extended horizontally and vertically, intersect at the aspiration point. This technique should only be used for large

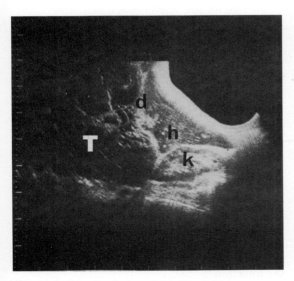

Fig. 14-3. Complex lesion above the right hemidiaphragm (d). Multiple loculated fluid areas are seen with extensive honeycomb of solid material (T). Below the diaphragm the liver (h) and right kidney (k) are seen.

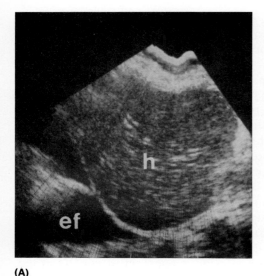

(A)

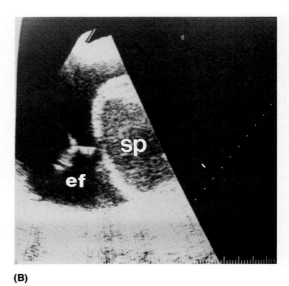

(B)

Fig. 14-4. **(A)** Right pleural effusion. A definite collection of fluid is seen (ef) below the right lung. Below the right hemidiaphragm, the liver (h) is seen. **(B)** Coronal scan with patient in decubitus position. The spleen (sp) is seen below the left hemidiaphragm. A large fluid collection (ef) is seen above the left hemidiaphragm.

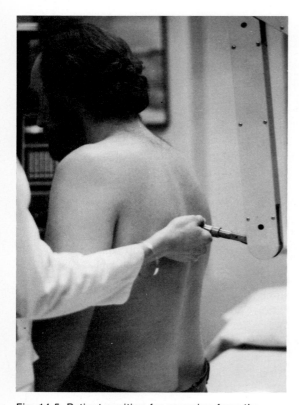

Fig. 14-5. Patient position for scanning from the posterior aspect for a pleural effusion.

effusions; small ones should be performed under precise ultrasound localization.

For a diagnostic thoracentesis, approximately 50 ml is ideally aspirated, and divided as follows:

0.5 ml for pH determination in a heparinised syringe

10 ml for LDH, protein and amylase in a chemistry tube

5 ml for bacteriology, for Gram stain and culture in a sterile tube

5 ml for cell count and differential in a hematology tube

The remainder of the sample is sent for cytology; as much as possible is required since the cells are concentrated by spinning and a large sample increases the chance of a positive yield.

A therapeutic tap is undertaken if there is a large amount of fluid which is causing dyspnea (difficulty in breathing). Frequently this results from heart failure or extensive tumor involvement of the pleura from primaries in the lung and breast.

The correlation between viscosity of the effusion and the ultrasound appearances is rather loose. In general, multiple echoes on the A-scan indicate many interfaces, while a

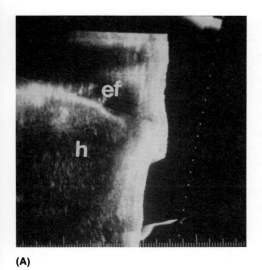

(A)

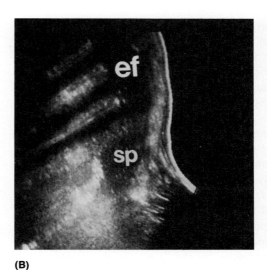

(B)

Fig. 14-6. **(A)** A right pleural effusion (ef) with the patient in the upright position. The liver (h) is seen below the right hemidiaphragm. **(B)** A left pleural effusion (ef) is seen with the patient in the upright position. The spleen (sp) is seen below the left hemidiaphragm.

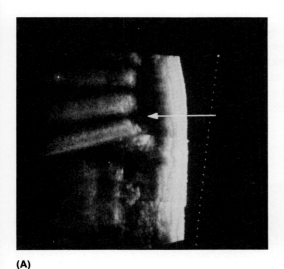

(A)

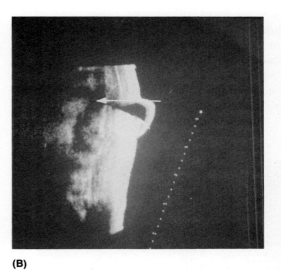

(B)

Fig. 14-7. **(A)** Pleural effusion (arrowed) before aspiration. **(B)** Post-aspiration scan showing smaller pleural effusion.

completely flat A-scan strongly suggests a simple liquid solution. However, recent blood clot may display virtually no interfaces and require a large bore needle, while a suspension of fairly small particles with significant echoes on the A-scan may be aspirated easily through a small needle. Because of these problems, in practice, it is appropriate to start with a small

bore needle, and if aspiration is difficult or impossible, to proceed to a large gauge bore.

RENAL CYST ASPIRATION

In recent years, the trend to puncture cystic renal lesions under fluoroscopic guidance has shifted to their precise localization and aspiration under ultrasound guidance. The primary advantages of this technique are the lack of patient exposure to ionizing radiation and the relative ease with which the procedure may be performed.

A renal mass is usually discovered by intravenous pyelography and the cystic nature of the mass established by subsequent ultrasound examination. Occasionally renal cysts may be large enough to be easily palpable. Renal cysts are common incidental findings and there is controversy over whether all of them should undergo cyst puncture. However, when the decision to aspirate a renal cyst has been made by the clinician, the patient is referred back to the ultrasound laboratory.

The sonographer must first ensure that a consent form has been completed and that the procedure has been explained to the patient. The standard consent form used for Radiologic procedures will be appropriate. The signed and witnessed consent form should be shown to the physician who will perform the procedure. The sonographer should also ascertain that the appropriate blood tests have been obtained, and that the results are available to the physician. Routine blood checks prior to aspiration and biopsy procedures consist of hemoglobin and hematocrit, prothrombin and bleeding time.

The procedure is initiated by scanning the kidney using the techniques described in the section on renal ultrasound (pp. 143–144). The lesion should be localized and evaluated for consistency before aspiration. The A-mode through the lesion is inspected with the B-scan transducer in contact with the skin over the lesion. A typical renal cyst and the corresponding A-mode are shown in Figure 14-8 A and B. The cyst should be visualized with the patient in the prone position. Aspiration should be performed with the patient in the prone position unless there is a specific obstacle preventing this. If an anterior approach is used, the needle traverses the peritoneal cavity and may pierce the gut before entering the cyst. In this way coliform organisms from the gut may be transmitted into the kidney and cause a renal abscess. The same disadvantage exists for a lateral approach in the decubitus position. When a skinny needle is used (23 gauge), the gut will not be significantly damaged by perforation, but it may result in bacterial contamination of the renal cyst. When larger needles are used,

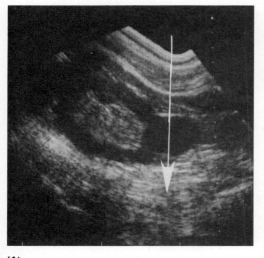

(A)

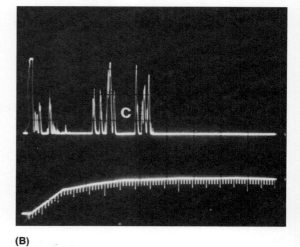

(B)

Fig. 14-8. **(A)** B-scan of left kidney showing large anechoic area in the lower pole. The arrow shows the position of the A-scan shown in Figure 15-8B. **(B)** A-scan showing completely echo free area due to the cyst (c).

puncture of the gut must be avoided, and this can be achieved most easily by a posterior approach, which avoids the peritoneal cavity.

The patient lies comfortably on the table with a small pillow under the abdomen to alleviate any inherent lordosis. With the patient in this position, the lesion is scanned and located precisely. Scans should be made in deep inspiration, total expiration and during normal breathing. The degree of movement of the lesion can be carefully monitored and positional changes noted. The physician performing the aspiration procedure marks the puncture site at an appropriate respiratory phase. The hub of a needle is useful for marking the skin surface, since other markers tend to be erased with sterilization of the skin. The angulation of the transducer should be noted and communicated to the physician, so that the needle can be similarly angulated.

When a cyst is large and virtually subcutaneous, needles can be easily inserted into it without the need to monitor the position of the needle during the procedure; the depth of the needle can be measured accurately from the B-scan. When smaller cysts or more deeply located ones are aspirated, continuing visualization of the needle is achieved using either a doughnut-shaped transducer or a slot transducer. An example of each is shown in Figure 14-9A and B.

The doughnut and slotted transducers are used in direct contact with the puncture site and consequently must be sterilized. Piezoelectric transducers to date may only be sterilized with gas (ethylene dioxide/CO_2) and this generally requires three to four days. The actual sterilization process is not this time consuming, but each package should receive a 48 to 72 hour incubation. When these transducers are employed, liberal amounts of Betadine may prove to be an adequate acoustic coupler. However, sterile mineral oil should be available if needed.

The use of real-time monitoring does not require sterilization, as the transducer head is not in direct contact with the operative field, but rather is at right angles to it on the patient's flank.

After the cyst is fully aspirated the char-

acter and volume of the contents is noted, and the fluid is placed in at least three tubes. These tubes are sent to the laboratory for cytology, biochemistry (fat and lactic dehydrogenase levels), and bacteriology. The cyst puncture

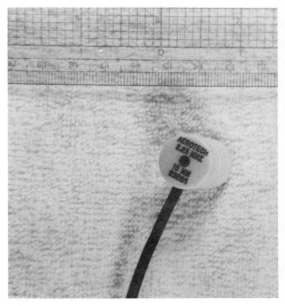

(A)

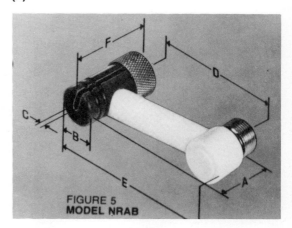

FIGURE 5
MODEL NRAB

(B)

Fig. 14-9. **(A)** Doughnut transducer, which can accomodate a needle down the central canal. **(B)** B-scan slot transducer. The aspiration needle can be passed down the center slot (C). The scanning arm can then be removed by slipping the needle out of the slot provided (Courtesy of K.B. Aerotech, Corp).

site should be rescanned and photographed at this time by conventional methods to re-examine the extent of the lesion and check for the possibility of any retained fluid. The wound is then protected with a small bandage. Renal cysts have a certain propensity for reaccumulation and ultrasound offers the best method for follow-up.

AMNIOCENTESIS

The use of high resolution, gray-scale ultrasound in obstetrics is documented in the chapter on obstetrical scanning (p. 55), and in the general literature. A further service available to the obstetrician is ultrasonic guidance of a needle into the uterine cavity to obtain a sample of amniotic fluid. Most frequently this is for the determination of the lecithin/sphingomyelin (L/S) ratio which is a reliable parameter of lung maturity. Other indications for amniocentesis include a genetic profile and determination of fetal sex when there is a family history of sex-linked disease, such as sickle cell disease and hemophilia. It is the sonographer's responsibility to localize the placenta and indicate an area which is free of placenta through which amniocentesis can be

carried out. This is especially important in patients with Rhesus incompatability; since if fetal blood should enter the maternal blood, it may induce production of antibodies. With high resolution, real-time machines, it is now easy to identify the insertion of the umbilical cord. This information is useful in the few cases where the placenta is entirely anterior so that no part of the uterine wall can be punctured without traversing the placenta. In these patients, it is important to identify the insertion of the umbilical cord and to direct the needle far away from this area through the edge of the placenta.

Technique

The gravid uterus is scanned in the sagittal and transverse planes. It is first determined whether the placenta is anterior or posterior. The fetal position is then determined, and an area is chosen which is both clear of placenta and of the fetus. The changing position of a very active fetus can be continuously monitored by real-time scanning. Indeed, amniocentesis can be monitored by the use of a real-time device scanning at right angles to the plane of the needle insertion. An area is cho-

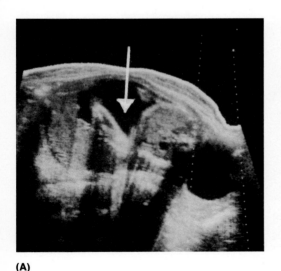

(A)

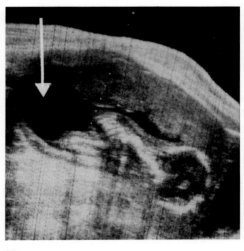

(B)

Fig. 14-10. **(A)** Posterior placenta. The arrow shows a suitable pocket of amniotic fluid for amniocentesis. **(B)** Anterior placenta, covering most of the anterior wall of the uterus. However, the arrow shows a suitable position, free of placenta, for amniocentesis.

sen which shows a generous collection of amniotic fluid. Figure 14-10A and B show examples of suitable sites for needle placement for amniocentesis. When possible, the lower uterine segment is avoided since the wall there is thicker and more difficult to penetrate. An anterior placenta generally requires a more lateral approach than a posterior placement. Ten milliliters of fluid are aspirated and placed in sterile collecting tubes for the necessary studies. After the fluid is aspirated the needle is withdrawn and the puncture site covered with a small bandage.

Equipment for Amniocentesis

Equipment necessary to perform amniocentesis is similar to that used for other aspiration and biopsy procedures. Table 14-1 shows the contents of the standard amniocentesis tray currently in use at this hospital. The physician who performs the tap should be asked for any specific requirements in addition to this tray.

TABLE 14-1. CONTENTS OF STANDARD AMNIOCENTESIS TRAY

Towels (sterile)
Clamps
Cotton
Gloves
Band-Aids (bandages)
Syringe: 3 cc.
Spinal needle
Needles: 19, 20 and 21 gauge
Test tube for fluid
Betadine
Lidocaine: 1%
Alcohol

TISSUE BIOPSY UNDER ULTRASONIC GUIDANCE

In recent years there has been a trend towards percutaneous biopsy procedures and away from exploratory laparotomy. This is particularly applicable for patients with apparently terminal illnesses, but in whom a definite diagnosis is required to exclude the possibility of a treatable lesion. Percutaneous biopsy can spare the patient unnecessary trauma of surgery.

The development of the skinny 23 gauge needle at Chiba University in Japan made such percutaneous biopsies possible and extremely safe. Skinny needle biopsy is impressive in that it is possible to traverse the gut with impunity to biopsy deep retroperitoneal organs such as the pancreas. The skinny needle is less thick than the suture needles used in surgery on the gut, which probably accounts for the extraordinary safety of these biopsy procedures (Fig. 14-11A and B). These needles are also extremely pliable, so that they bend freely when inserted into an organ which moves with respiration, without lacerating the organ. However, the yield is in terms of isolated cells rather than specimens of tissue; that is, cytology rather than histology. This certainly compromises the pathological accuracy of skinny needle biopsy as a diagnostic pro-

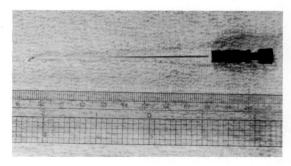

(A)

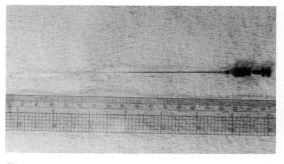

(B)

Fig. 14-11. **(A)** Lumbar puncture needle, gauge 18, used for amniocentesis and thoracentesis. **(B)** Chiba 'skinny' needle, gauge 23. Note that this is nearly twice as long as the lumbar puncture needle.

cedure, and in large series of patients, successful biopsies were obtained in just over 70 percent of patients with retroperitoneal malignancies. Nevertheless, this is an impressive number of patients for whom pathological diagnosis can be made, and for whom exploratory surgery is unnecessary.

Technique

A retroperitoneal lesion is identified by transverse and longitudinal scanning in the usual way. The preliminary blood work and signed consent forms are checked. A suitable site for biopsy is chosen by the physician, clear of any blood vessels or overlying gut. A photograph is taken of the elected biopsy area with calipers superimposed on the proposed biopsy site. This site is marked on the skin by indentation produced by firm pressure from the hub of the needle. The distance from the skin surface to the desired depth in the tumor is measured. The skin is sterilized with Betadine and infiltrated with 1 percent lidocaine. It is our custom to place an intramuscular needle through the skin and rectus abdominis sheath to provide a firm channel through these tough layers for the very pliable skinny needle. The skinny needle is then passed through to the depth identified from the scans, and firm aspiration into a syringe containing normal sterile saline is attempted, while several small cuts are made with the needle into the tumor tissue. The contents of the needle are then ejected onto a slide and immediately fixed with "Spray-cyte." The aspirate remaining in the syringe is placed into containers and sent for cytology. The procedure is repeated three or four times, and all aspirated material and slides are sent to cytology. In addition, the syringe is sent since this can be washed out, and the resulting material spun down to make a cell block.

Because of the limitations imposed by obtaining cells rather than pieces of tissue, many of our referring physicians prefer the use of a routine liver biopsy needle, rather than the skinny needle. Obviously this can only be used in an organ such as the liver, where there is no question of gut or other vis-

cus intervening between the skin and the tumor site. However, when tumor is clearly seen in the left lobe of the liver by ultrasound, it is perverse to biopsy the right lobe of the liver purely for the sake of routine. Under these circumstances when the lesion can be identified in the left lobe, the overlying skin is marked and the angle of approach approximated, as well as the distance from other structures. Such an ultrasonically guided biopsy from the scan shown in Figure 14-12 revealed an adenocarcinoma of the pancreas from a primary tumor well demonstrated by ultrasound.

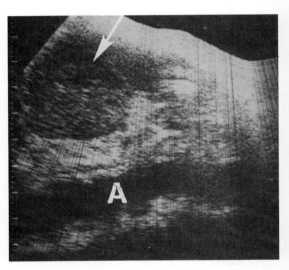

Fig. 14-12. Left lobe of the liver anterior to the aorta (A). A very subtle lesion is seen arrowed. The arrow also shows the position and direction for biopsy using a standard Klatskin liver biopsy needle. Ultrasound visualization allows the great vessels to be avoided by this large cutting needle. Biopsy of this lesion revealed adenocarcinoma, and the primary in the pancreas was well visualized in the tail of the pancreas by ultrasound.

CONCLUSION

Needle aspiration and biopsy procedures under ultrasound visualization are rapidly becoming well accepted techniques for obtaining both fluid and cells for diagnostic purposes. Although computerized tomography is also used for the same purpose, the wide availability and access to ultrasound machines makes this a more logical modality for guidance. Persuaded by the apparent safety of aspiration techniques using skinny needles, a rapid increase in the use of such techniques appears to be inevitable.

SUGGESTED READING

Editorial: Utility of needle aspiration of tumours. Br Med J, 1507-1508, Jn 19, 1978.

Haaga JR, Alfidi RJ: Precise biopsy localization by computed tomography. Radiology 118:603-607, 1976.

Hancke S, Holm HH, Kock F: Ultrasonically guided percutaneous fine needle biopsy of the pancreas. Surg Gynecol Obstet 140:361-364, 1975.

Holm HH, Als O, Gammelgaard J: Percutaneous aspiration and biopsy procedures under ultrasound visualization. In: Clinics in Diagnostic Ultrasound, Vol. 1, New York, Churchill Livingstone, 1979.

Lalli AF, McCormack LJ, Zelch M, et al: Aspiration biopsies of chest lesions. Radiology 127:35-40, 1978.

McLoughlin MJ, Lander B, McHattie J, et al: Fine needle aspiration biopsy of malignant lesions in and around the pancreas. Cancer 41:2413-2419, 1978.

Rasmussen SN, Holm HH, Kristensen JK, et al: Ultrasonically guided liver biopsy. Br Med J 2:500-502, 1972.

Sanders RC: Percutaneous punctures: a new radiological skill. Radiology 127:883-834, 1978.

Sherlock P, Kim YS, Koss LG: Cytologic diagnosis of cancer from aspirated material obtained at liver biopsy. Am J Dig Dis 12:396, 1967.

15

Water Bath Scanning
and Special Examinations

RALPH WINTERS

INTRODUCTION

When the early pioneers explored the potential uses of pulsed-wave, high frequency ultrasound in medicine, there were problems in attaining an acoustic coupling between the large transducers in use and the body. This was initially solved by scanning the patient in a water tank. Several early attempts at utilizing this concept for total body scanning produced high quality scans, but the technique proved to be rather cumbersome and was subsequently abandoned. There are, however, definite advantages in the use of a water bath, and more and more systems are now utilizing this principle. These advantages have been considered (pp. 29–31) and are summarized as follows: the organ to be imaged can be placed in the focal zone of the transducer so that the complex near field lies in the water bath; large transducers can be used, which can be more highly focused; and difficulties in maintaining

contact over irregular skin surfaces are eliminated because a soft water bag conforms to the body contour.

The major disadvantage of water bath scanning is the occurrence of reverberations (see pp. 35–37). These can be overcome if the transducer is the same distance from the skin as the depth of the tissue which is to be imaged. The reverberation is then beyond the area of interest. Alternatively, in commercially available systems, the fluid has been matched to the transducer which prevents the occurrence of any reverberations at all (pp. 30–31).

The water bath presently in use is quite simple in design and construction. It may be purchased or constructed to suit individual needs. Two possible configurations for water baths are shown in Figure 15-1. In designing a water bath, foresight will allow for an opening large enough to accomodate a linear array real-time scanning head. In addi-

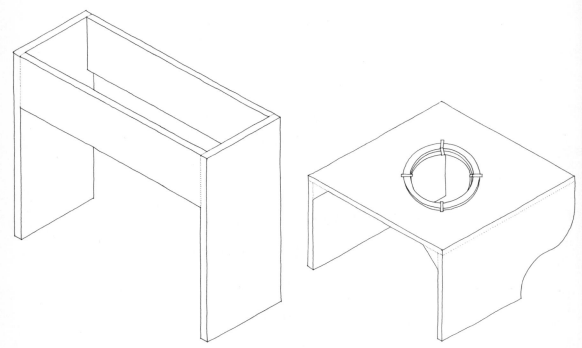

Fig. 15-1. Frames for simple water baths which can be purchased, or constructed in the laboratory. (Courtesy Rob Charney.)

tion to a water bath, a bag of air-free, normal saline should be kept available. This may be particularly useful in assessing chest wall thickness.

APPLICATIONS OF WATER BATH SCANNING

Thyroid

Normal Anatomy The normal adult thyroid is a bilobed organ, joined together anteriorly by tissue called the isthmus. It weighs between 15 to 35 grams in the adult and is draped around the trachea at the level of the fourth to sixth cervical vertebrae (Fig. 15-2). The entire organ is enclosed in fascia and partially covered by the sternomastoid and strap neck muscles. On the posterior-lateral aspect of each lobe the parathyroid glands are located, which occasionally undergo enlargement due to hyperplasia or tumor. The thyroid and parathyroid glands are vital in the regulation of metabolic function. The thyroid controls the

metabolic rate through its released hormones, thyroxin and triiodothyronine. Both these contain iodine which is taken up from the blood and concentrated by the thyroid. Both the thyroid, through the action of its hormone calcitonin, and the parathyroid, through the action of the hormone parathormone, are important in the regulation of calcium metabolism.

Pathology The two methods used for imaging the thyroid are isotope imaging (using [99m]technetium pertechnetate, I[131], I[123]) and ultrasound. These methods are complementary, since isotope imaging indicates the functional activity of the gland while ultrasound images the structural components. The most common clinical problem is the management of a thyroid nodule. Initially, the patient is referred for nuclear scanning, since most malignancies and all innocent cysts do not take up iodine. Thus, the patient with a "cold" area on the isotope scan may be referred for ultrasound scanning to differentiate between a solid and cystic lesion. Thyroid cysts are easily differentiated by

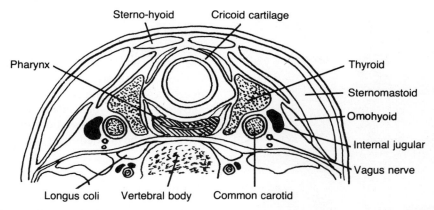

Sterno-hyoid   Cricoid cartilage

Pharynx

Thyroid

Sternomastoid

Omohyoid

Internal jugular

Vagus nerve

Longus coli   Vertebral body   Common carotid

Fig. 15-2. Schema of cross-section of the neck, at the level of the cricoid cartilage. The lateral lobes of the thyroid are seen in the paratracheal position, covered by the sternomastoid and strap muscles. Note the position of the great vessels posterior and lateral to the lateral lobes of the thyroid.

ultrasound. At the present time, there appears to be no definite means of distinguishing whether a solid lesion is benign or malignant based on the ultrasound appearances. Eighty percent of these solid lesions are benign. However, if multiple solid abnormalities are seen on ultrasound, the disease is more likely to be benign. Many patients with low clinical suspicion of malignancy are placed on suppression therapy, and they are referred back for ultrasound examination to determine whether therapy has resulted in any change in the size of the tumor. Thus, serial ultrasound studies may be more valuable than a single study. If a lesion continues to grow despite suppression therapy, surgical intervention must be considered. If the lesion decreases in size, this is reassuring for conservative clinical management.

Ultrasound Scanning Technique The thyroid may be examined by ultrasound in two separate ways: by direct contact scanning or through a water bath. Generally speaking, the water bath produces more consistent, higher quality results. Simple sector contact scanning is compromised by variations in skin contour, especially in the transverse plane, and compound scanning may obscure small lesions. Water bath scanning, however, is quite simple and good results are routinely obtained.

The patient is placed in the supine posi-

tion and the neck slightly hyperextended by placing a rolled towel behind the patient's neck. Mineral oil or acoustic gel is applied between the water bath and the patient's neck. The contents of the water bath can be degassed easily, by leaving the fluid in the lab for a period of time. When the water bath is placed on the patient's neck, care should be taken to ensure that no air is trapped between the bag and the skin surface (Fig. 15-3). Gentle pressure from within the bag helps to displace any small air pockets. The depth of the water is adjusted so that the thyroid is in the focal zone of the transducer and the reverberation is beyond the area of interest. A short focused transducer at 3.5 MHz or 5 MHz can be utilized. The TGC should be delayed so that it does not start within the water bath, but at the skin surface.

The thyroid gland is scanned in both transverse and longitudinal planes. Normal thyroid scans are shown in Figure 15-4A and B. Since ultrasound is a tomographic technique, multiple sections must be taken to ensure that the largest diameter of a lesion has been imaged for comparative measurements. The neck should be palpated by the sonographer and ultrasonologist to ensure that the suspicious area has been imaged. The isotopic scans should be provided for the interpreting physician so that a combined report can be made.

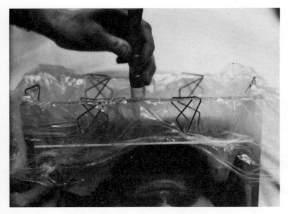

Fig. 15-3. Water bath in position for thyroid scanning.

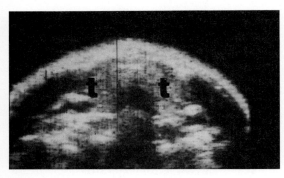

(A)

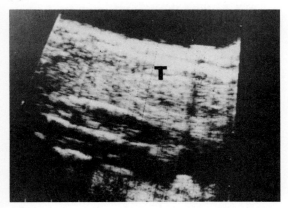

(B)

Fig. 15-4. **(A)** Transverse scan of the thyroid. The lateral lobes of the thyroid (t) are seen on either side of the trachea. **(B)** Longitudinal scan of the thyroid (T). The carotid artery (c) is seen posteriorly.

Thyroid cysts are easily imaged by ultrasound and one example is shown in Figure 15-5A and B; a solid lesion is shown in Figure 15-6, which proved to be an adenoma. Commonly, there is evidence for central necrosis within an adenoma. Figure 15-7 shows a similar solid lesion which is entirely uniform in its ultrasound appearances, yet proved to be a medullary carcinoma of the thyroid.

Baker's Cysts

Bursal or Baker's cysts are serosanguinous fluid collections in the bursa of the knee, dissecting in varying degrees to the lower extremities. They may be multiloculated and are often associated with degenerative bone disease, especially rheumatoid arthritis. Occasionally, they have small solid components known as "melon seeds." While contact scanning problems are not acute in the examination of the lower extremities, a water bath is useful to improve scan quality, especially in the patient with reduced mobility due to advanced arthritic changes. The actual scanning technique is the same as that previously described for the thyroid. In scanning Baker's cysts, both legs should be scanned to provide comparative data for interpretation. Scans of a Baker's cyst and normal extremity are shown below (Fig. 15-8A and B).

Indications for Water Bath Scanning of the Abdomen

There are numerous situations in scanning the abdomen when utilization of a water bath greatly aids in achieving technically satisfactory scans. While each is unique and subject to variations in application, a general discussion of these uses is of value.

The question of non-shadowing gallstones may be resolved by the use of a stand-off water bath. A litre bag of normal saline, "burped" free of air, will serve well. It has been shown that calculi outside the focal plane of the transducer may fail to cast the typical acoustical shadow (p. 119). This is especially true when a long, focused transducer is used to

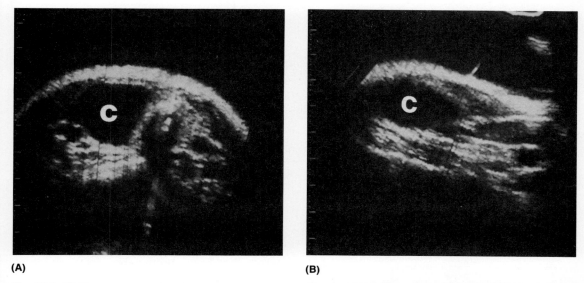

(A)   **(B)**

Fig. 15-5. **(A)** Transverse section through the neck showing the thyroid cyst (c). **(B)** Longitudinal scan showing thyroid cyst (c).

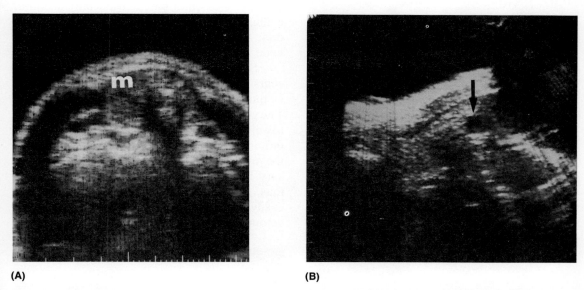

(A)   **(B)**

Fig. 15-6. **(A)** Transverse scan of thyroid showing large, predominantly solid mass (m) in the right lateral lobe. This proved to be an adenoma. **(B)** Longitudinal scan; adenomas may show small areas of central necrosis (arrowed).

image a superficial gallbladder. By employing a water bath, the transducer is backed away from the gallbladder to a plane which allows the calculi to fall into the focal zone. Examples of this phenomenon are demonstrated (Fig. 15-9A and B). The same effect may be achieved by changing from a long to a medium focused transducer. However, at smaller facilities, this choice may not always be available.

The post-surgical patient is an excellent candidate for water bath scanning. Often the field of interest is compromised by scar tissue, wounds, bandages, sutures, etc. Sterile oil is placed around the area and the water bath applied in the usual manner. This allows the sonographer to get as close as possible to the scanning area with a minimal amount of discomfort to the patient. The technique may be exceptionally helpful in delineating small areas of pus formation around a wound, that would otherwise be inaccessible.

Young children may be scanned with a water bath to ensure high quality scans. Contact scanning may be disrupted by frequent movement, and continued applications of the transducer to the skin aggravates an infirm child, making it quite difficult to complete the

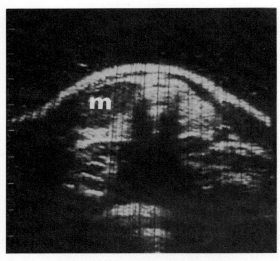

Fig. 15-7. Transverse scan of the neck showing a solid lesion, entirely uniform throughout, but which proved to be a medullary carcinoma (m).

examination. However, applying a WARM bath to the abdomen is a one-time procedure, and, it, accompanied by reduced lighting and subdued conversational tone, enables the sonographer to achieve repeated scans with a minimum of distress. In addition, the quality of the scans will certainly be improved.

The post-radical mastectomy patient may be referred by the radiation therapist for evaluation of chest-wall thickness prior to initiating radiation therapy. Such a patient can be very difficult to scan, and a water bath alleviates many of the problems. The potential radiation therapy port should be marked out on the skin prior to the examination. Either the standard water bath or a bag of saline is placed across the chest, and the area is scanned in as many planes as necessary to achieve a realistic contour map of the chest. This should be accomplished with the patient assuming the identical position to be used during radiation therapy. The water bath is especially useful in evaluating the axilla, and some work has been done with this technique in delineating lymph node involvement.

Scanning of the testicles and penis presents problems to the sonographer which may be quickly resolved by the use of a water bath. The genitalia are supported from below with a towel and liberally covered with acoustic gel or mineral oil. The water bath is placed across the area of interest and scanned in the necessary fashion. High quality scans of seminomas, and other testicular abnormalities are easily obtained in this fashion with a minimal amount of discomfort to the patient.

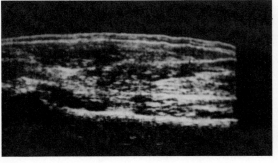

(A)

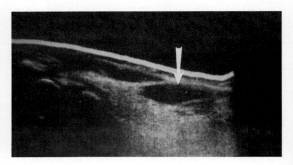

(B)

Fig. 15-8. Longitudinal scans of leg from the posterior surface. **(A)** Normal patient; **(B)** An elongated, fluid filled, superificial mass is seen, consistent with a Baker's cyst (arrowed).

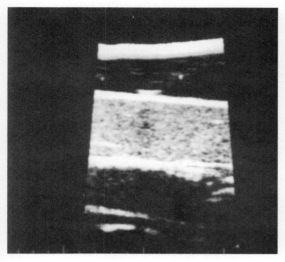
(A)

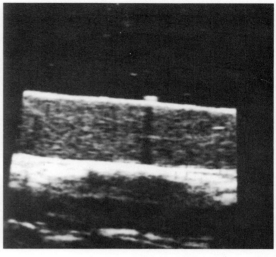
(B)

Fig. 15-9. **(A)** Scan of gallstone on a tissue phantom, when the gallstone is in the near zone of the transducer with a wide beamwidth. Note that there is no evidence of an acoustic shadow. **(B)** Scan of gallstone lying on a tissue phantom, showing well marked shadowing when the stone is situated in the focal zone of the transducer.

Finally, water bath scanning is a tremendous aid in obtaining high quality specimen scans *in vitro*. All personnel involved in ultrasound should, at one time or another, want to correlate specimens with their ultrasound appearances. We have tried several techniques to achieve this, but none has worked as well as the water bath technique. The specimen is placed on the table and covered with liberal amounts of oil. The water bath is placed over the organ and excellent images can be obtained. This also prevents direct contact of the scanning apparatus and the specimen. Examples of these are shown below (Fig. 15-10A and B).

While the examples which we have mentioned represent some of the uses for water bath scanning, they are by no means all inclusive. The water bath is a tool that the sonographer must learn to use and apply as individual situations dictate. With the advent of high quality, linear array, real-time transducers, the size of the scanning head often makes it difficult to maintain skin contact. Here again, the water bath has been helpful in eliminating scanning problems. More uses will certainly arise, and an awareness of the potential appli-

cations of the water bath will help the sonographer obtain scans that would otherwise be impossible to achieve.

SPECIAL EXAMINATIONS

Prostate

The prostate is a firm, echogenic organ, located at the base of the bladder in males, and frequently produces problems in patients over 50 years of age. The urethra, which conveys urine from the bladder out of the body, passes through the center of the prostate. A common result of prostatic disease is hydronephrosis and hydroureter. Benign prostatic hypertrophy (BPH) affects a large number of elderly men, and the degree of prostate enlargement as well as response to treatment can be quickly assessed with current ultrasound equipment. Patients may also be referred to ultrasound after the discovery of metastatic disease, for investigation of possible primary tumor. Ninety-six percent of all tumors involving the prostate are adenocarcinomas; 80 percent of these metastasize to the bone, and

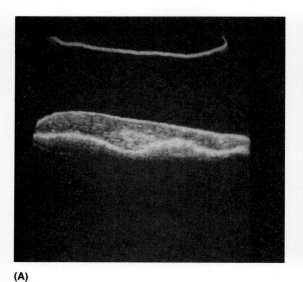

(A)

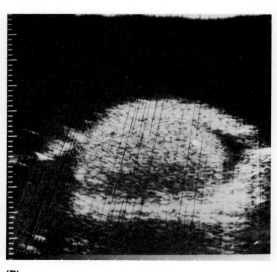

(B)

Fig. 15-10. In vitro scanning of pathological specimens. **(A)** Longitudinal scan of an excised pancreas showing the typical echogenic structure of the normal parenchyma. **(B)** Scan of a dermoid showing echogenic mass with high attenuation causing some loss of amplitude distally. This is the so-called 'tip of the iceberg' sign.

very infrequently the liver may also be involved.

Technique The prostate must be scanned with a full urinary bladder, in the same way as the standard OB/GYN patient. The examination should be initiated with midline longitudinal sections through the lower pelvis. From the longitudinal sections, an angle which allows the transducer to be perpendicular to the true axis of the prostate can be chosen. The arm is then rotated 90 degrees and transverse scans obtained. The extreme inferior-posterior location of the prostate makes it impossible to obtain adequate transverse scans without employing this angulation into the pelvis.

Radiographically, the prostate is an ex-tremely difficult organ to visualize successfully. This is an especially difficult problem for the radiation dosimetrist, who must develop an acceptable radiation therapy treatment plan. The method in the past has been to fill the bulb of a standard Foley catheter with mercury and allow it to drape the prostate, thereby providing a contour profile. With ultrasound, the catheter can be filled with a small amount of barium and the exact center of the prostate ascertained. The organ-to-skin distance, as well as the relationship to surrounding organs can be accurately profiled. Though not currently in wide practice, this is an excellent technique which provides the radiation dosimetrist with a wealth of vital information.

16

Neurosonography

RALPH WINTERS

INTRODUCTION

Echoencephalography is an excellent, non-invasive, diagnostic tool for both emergency room and general medical use. It is especially valuable in those hospitals without easy access to computerized axial tomography. Its major value is to identify the patient with a space-occupying intracranial lesion, which may require immediate surgical intervention. It is also a valuable complementary technique to [99m]technetium brain scanning and for ruling out tumors as a cause of certain organic brain disorders and psychiatric disturbances. The method is also useful in assessing ventricular size when hydrocephalus is suspected.

Anatomy

To perform echoencephalography a good knowledge of the intracranial anatomy and the ventricular system in particular is needed. The brain contains a complex system of fluid-filled structures known as the ventricular system. This is intricate in shape and is shown schematically in Figure 16-1. The two lateral ventricles lie to either side of the midline and are divided into frontal, occipital and temporal horns, according to the lobes of the brain they penetrate. The lateral ventricles communicate with the third ventricle by means of the Foramen of Monroe. The third ventricle is smaller than the lateral ones occupying a slit-like space between the inner aspects of the thalami. It is an important structure to be identified on the A-mode echoencephalograph as well as in the estimation of the biparietal diameters. The third ventricle is continuous posteriorly with a slender tube which runs into the pons and medulla of the brain and is known as the Aqueduct of Sylvius. In the angle between the medulla and the cerebellum, this aquaduct opens into the fourth ventricle.

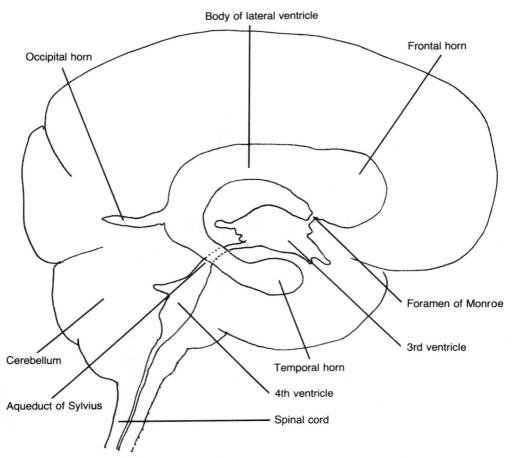

Fig. 16-1. Sagittal section of the brain showing the ventricular system. The third ventricle can be traced through the Foramen of Monroe (interventricular foramen) into the large lateral ventricles. The lateral and third ventricles contain the choroid plexus from which the cerebrospinal fluid is produced. The third ventricle is continuous with the fourth ventricle through the Aqueduct of Sylvius which passes through the midbrain.

The ventricular system is filled with clear cerebro-spinal fluid (CSF) which is produced by the choroid plexus, mainly in the lateral ventricles. This fluid drains into the fourth ventricle and escapes through medial and lateral foramens (of Magendie and Luschka). The fluid is then in the subarachnoid space and circulates freely over the surface of the brain. The fluid is mainly reabsorbed in the large venous sinuses which lie on the inner surfaces of the skull.

The brain is enclosed and protected by three membranous sheaths known as the pia mater, arachnoid mater and dura mater. The pia mater is in intimate contact with the brain and extends deeply into its convolutions. The arachnoid mater passes across the pia mater leaving a potential gap known as the subarachnoid space. The arachnoid is so named due to its resemblance to a spider, in that thin strands of tissue cross the subarachnoid space. The CSF drains into the subarachnoid space, bathing the brain in nutrients and providing a water jacket for the brain which reduces the effects of trauma. Arteries supplying the brain travel through this space and may bleed and cause a subarachnoid hemorrhage. A congenital defect in the arterial wall predisposes to aneurysm formation which may rupture and cause such hemorrhage.

Fused with the periosteum of the inner skull table is the dura mater. It is a tough fibrous membrane which folds deeply between the two cerebral hemispheres to form the cerebral falx. The falx cerebri is easily identified ultrasonically within the fetal skull. The dura mater produces two potential spaces, the extra-dural and subdural. Both are sites of intracranial hemorrhage with the subdural being the most frequent. In terms of vascular involvement, it should be remembered that arteries lie in the subarachnoid space; cerebral veins occupy the subdural space; and the meningeal arteries, supplying the red bone marrow of the skull, lie in the extradural space.

Pathology

Encapsulation of the brain by a rigid bony skeleton leads to unique and life threatening emergencies as a result of any space-occupying lesion. Since the brain is prevented from expanding, pressure builds up within the skull and produces malfunctions, characterized by reduced level of consciousness, coma, paralysis and eventual death. It is this progressive syndrome which the sonographer is often called upon to evaluate. The detection of a midline shift through the use of A-mode echoencephalography may facilitate the institution of life-saving surgical intervention.

An arterial bleed results in blood mixing with the CSF and flowing into the subarachnoid space. This is a subarachnoid hemorrhage and offers dramatic signs and symptoms. Headache, nausea, vomiting and shifting degrees of consciousness may all occur depending on the extent of the bleed. Lumbar puncture in these patients reveals blood-stained CSF. Since blood passes freely into the subarachnoid space, there is no localized hematoma and no brain compression. Therefore, these patients have a normal echoencephalograph but display signs of an intracranial catastrophe.

Ultrasound is of great aid in the diagnosis of a subdural hematoma. A subdural hematoma is often a slowly accumulating lesion, characteristically occurring in the elderly patient

with a prior history of a minor skull trauma. These patients exhibit progressive deterioration of their mental faculties, often attributed to senility and resulting in long-term nursing internment or prolonged psychiatric evaluation. The condition may worsen until death ensues, making it an essential echoencephalographic diagnosis.

The extradural hematoma is the most lethal and the most treatable of intracranial hemorrhages. It is the result of a bleeding meningeal artery and is sometimes accompanied by skull fracture. Detection of an extradural bleed is a major reason for close observations of patients with head injuries. Unless recognized at an early stage, this condition may result in rapid deterioration and death. There is seldom time to transfer a patient to a center for computerized axial tomography. A-mode evaluation for mid-line shift is quite sensitive in detecting an extradural hematoma and can give the diagnosis which will allow life-saving surgical intervention.

One of the most common types of intracranial hemorrhage is the cerebral vascular accident (CVA) or stroke. It is due to a hemorrhage actually within the brain substance and may lead to varying degrees of paralysis. Occasionally, hematomas may form which are detectable as a midline shift.

In addition to hematomas, other space occupying lesions, such as primary and metastatic tumors, may be suspected in patients referred for ultrasonic evaluation. If the sonographer demonstrates a repeatable shift of the midline structures, regardless of origin, the neurologist is quickly alerted to the fact that some brain compression is occurring and may take appropriate action.

TECHNIQUE

The examination is best performed with the patient in the supine position and the sonographer seated at the patient's head (Fig. 16-2). Although the examination may be conducted with both the examiner and patient seated, the supine approach allows the sonographer's arm to rest on the stretcher alongside the patient's

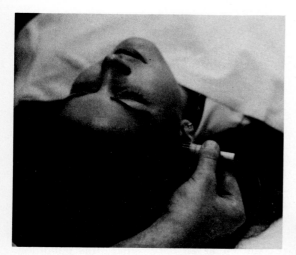

Fig. 16-2. Correct placement of the transducer to image the ventricles in the midline complex.

be employed. If the available unit does not have TGC display, it may have been preset by the manufacturer and should be obtained from their representatives. Care should be exercised not to extend the slope so far as to preclude the adequate display of a potential near field midline shift. This slope is only useful when the near wall anatomy is not of interest. After the TGC is set, it may be turned off so that

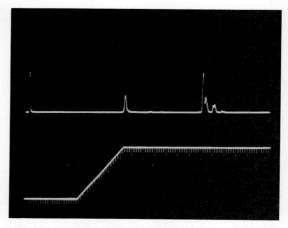

Fig. 16-3. TGC setting for determining the midline position. An initial delay reduces the near field echoes, while the knee of the curve is broken just before the midline echoes.

head and prevents involuntary movement or fatigue to the operator's arm.

Several opinions have been expressed with regard to the placement of the transducer on the patient's head. In the author's experience, there are no definite rules, because of the major variations which exist in the normal contour of the parietal bones. Since a frequency of 1.6 or 2.25 MHz is employed with adults, the transducer face is usually rather wide, and this also precludes exact placement of the beam. The transducer is placed just anterior and a little superior to the external auditory meatus and gently rocked to permit necessary structure identification.

Hair contains considerable air and makes adequate coupling especially difficult. Generous quantities of ultrasound gel are used. The examination commences with placement of the transducer on the right side of the head. Conventionally, this projection is shown on the top of the Polaroid (Fig. 16-3). The transducer is slowly rocked until the midline of the brain is identified as well as the far wall complex. At this time the TGC is adjusted into a steep ramp just before the midline echo (as shown in photo). If a known lesion is to be evaluated, the slope of the curve must be appropriately set and either opposite wall evaluation or a near field standoff technique should

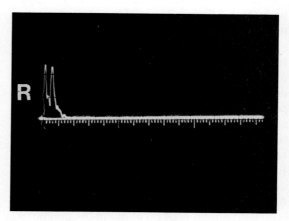

Fig. 16-4. With the transducer in contact with the right side of the head, the initial pulse is seen from the near side of the skull and the examination commences.

only the straight centimeter scale is shown (Fig. 16-4). The TGC remains in effect, even though it is not displayed.

When performing midline echoencephalography, the most reliable landmark is the third ventricle. Its size and characteristic pulsations of the base line make it unique in appearance. Four factors affect the A-mode characteristics of the third ventricle. The two mechanical factors are the degree of beam focusing and the frequency employed. The two physiological parameters are the width of the ventricle and possibly the pressure of the CSF within it. Adjustment of the overall gain control, after the third ventricle has been identified, eliminates electronic noise from the baseline. If the unit is equipped with a reject control, it is also useful for fine noise control.

Attention is now directed to the far wall complex. Depending again on the mechanical factors employed and the densities of the skull tables, this may also vary slightly in appearance. However, a three-pronged trident is often identified. When the midline and the far wall are suitably displayed, the first exposure of the Polaroid is made so that the upper tracing always indicates the right to left transducer position. The f-stop of the camera should be adjusted to allow three exposures on a single Polaroid without over saturating the film. The tracing is now inverted, using the available switch. This is normally labelled with a capital A and an inverted V. The exam is repeated now with the transducer placed on the left side of the head and the result is photographed. The lower tracing always represents the left to right study.

Some echoencephalography units provide outlets for two tranducers, one of which will act only as a receiver. With transducers placed on either side of the head, the unit then electronically divides the distance between the two transducer faces and gives the appropriate midline measurement on the screen. The use of a theoretical midline has been much debated. If performed in the beginning of an examination, it may prejudice a novice examiner. It also presupposes that the measurement is at the same point as the ventricular measurement. However, when done last, it can be

a useful indicator as to whether the exam will hold up to careful validation.

An innovation to midline echoencephalograpy is the midliner echoencephlograph. Transducer placement parameters remain the same. However with the computerized unit, the midline is determined automatically and any degree of shift is instantly calculated and displayed on a bar graph. This instrument removes the need for much operator expertise and is beneficial for non-specialized personnel who are performing echoencephalography. However, its application to other A-mode investigative techniques has been sacrificed (Fig. 16-5).

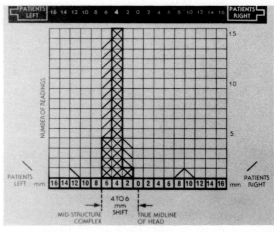

Fig. 16-5. Computerized A-mode echoencephalograph. A histogram is constructed of the midline position. The midline echoes derived from both sides coincide and there is no sign of shift of the midline structures.

VALIDATION AND INTERPRETATION OF MIDLINE ECHOENCEPHALOGRAPHY

Validation of an echoencephalograph does not tell the examiner whether or not pathology exists. It does, however, tell him that the structures examined in both the right to left, and left to right tracing, are in the same original position. A measurement is made from the right side of the head to the center of the ventricular complex. When both walls of the ventricle are defined, be sure to measure from the

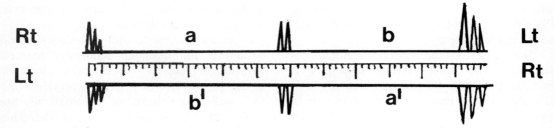

Fig. 16-6. Echoencephalogram. The upper tracing shows the position of the midline as determined from the right side of the head. The lower line shows the position as determined from the left. Notice that b and b¹ and a and a¹ should be equal. The midline echoes should be perfectly superimposed when the skull tables are aligned. ·

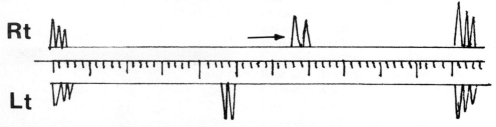

Fig. 16-7. Abnormal echoencephalogram showing a shift of the midline. The midline complex is shifted towards the left on both tracings, indicating a right-sided, space-occupying lesion. Notice that the difference between the midline complexes is twice the midline shift.

beginning of each detection to assess the true midline accurately. This measurement is termed the *a measurement*. Using a pair of calipers, this distance is transferred to the bottom, using the center of the ventricle as a starting point and is called *a'*. The procedure is reversed, using the L-middle bottom measurement as *b* and its equivalent on the top as *b'*. If the two outer marks align, the examination is valid and may be interpreted. However, poor alignment of the inner skull tables is an indication of unequal transducer placement and is a quick general guide to validity (Fig. 16-6).

An example of an abnormal echoencephalograph is shown below (Fig. 16-7). The distance between the two midline complexes is measured, and that value is divided by two. Value is the real distance the ventricle has been displaced off the midline. Up to a 3 mm shift should be considered within normal limits, due to variations in cranial symmetry. The direction of the shift is always from the greater to the lesser distance. For example, in the photograph below (Fig. 16-7) the greatest transducer/midline distance is on the right, making this a right to left shift with the lesion located on the right side of the head. If the examination is considered to be positive, it is often helpful to do several studies and confirm the accuracy of your findings.

HYDROCEPHALUS

Hydrocephalus refers to a condition characterized by obstruction to the ventricular system with subsequent dilatation of the ventricles. It is essentially a condition noted in neonates and a frequent accompaniment of meningitis, secondary to spina bifida. In neonates, this condition may be diagnosed with the techniques described above. The newborn skull may also be contact scanned or scanned in a water bath in gray-scale, using the B-mode. This is an especially effective technique for revealing the continual success or failure of ventricular shunts. However, another form

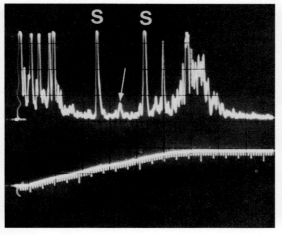

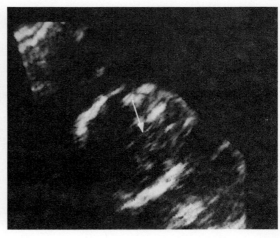

(A)   **(B)**

Fig. 16-8. **(A)** A-scan through the fetal head showing the midline (arrowed) and skull table (S). **(B)** B-scan of 18 week fetus showing midline (arrowed) with the lateral ventricles on either side.

of ventricular evaluation may be performed on the fetus, in vitro. This technique utilizes a combination of B-mode contact scanning and simultaneous A-mode assessment. While a sonographer is performing a routine obstetrical examination, the ability to recognize and quantitate the size of the lateral ventricles is clinically important. When the angle of asynclitism has been established and the arm correctly placed for obtaining the biparietal diameter, an accurate estimation of ventricular width may be made. The ventricles appear on the B-mode scan as sonolucent areas lying to either side of the falx cerebri. The B-mode transducer is placed on either side of the maternal abdomen and the corresponding A-mode reviewed (Fig. 16-8A and B). This information is vital to successful prenatal diagnosis of hydrocephaly.

In conclusion, echoencephalography is a proven, reliable, effective and low cost tool for distinguishing a wide variety of intracranial conditions.

SUGGESTED READING

White DN, Hudson AC: The future of A-mode echoencephalography. The development of automated techniques. Neurology 21:140-153, 1971.

White DN, Hanna LF: Automatic midline echoencephalography. Examination of 3333 consecutive cases with an automatic midline computer. Neurology 24:230-252, 1971.

McKinney WM, Toole JF, Sharp WT: Evaluation of 500 psychiatric inpatients by midline echoencephalography. Acta Radiol 5:865-870, 1966.

Brown R: Analysis of echoencephalograms. Neurology 18:237-242, 1968.

Goldberg B: Head and neck. In Goldberg BB, Kotler MN, Ziskin MC, Waxham RD (Eds): Diagnostic Uses of Ultrasound. New York, Grune & Stratton, 1977, pp 70-114.

Index

Page Numbers In Italics Represent Illustrations